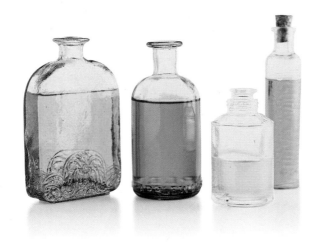

aroma remedies

chrissy wildwood

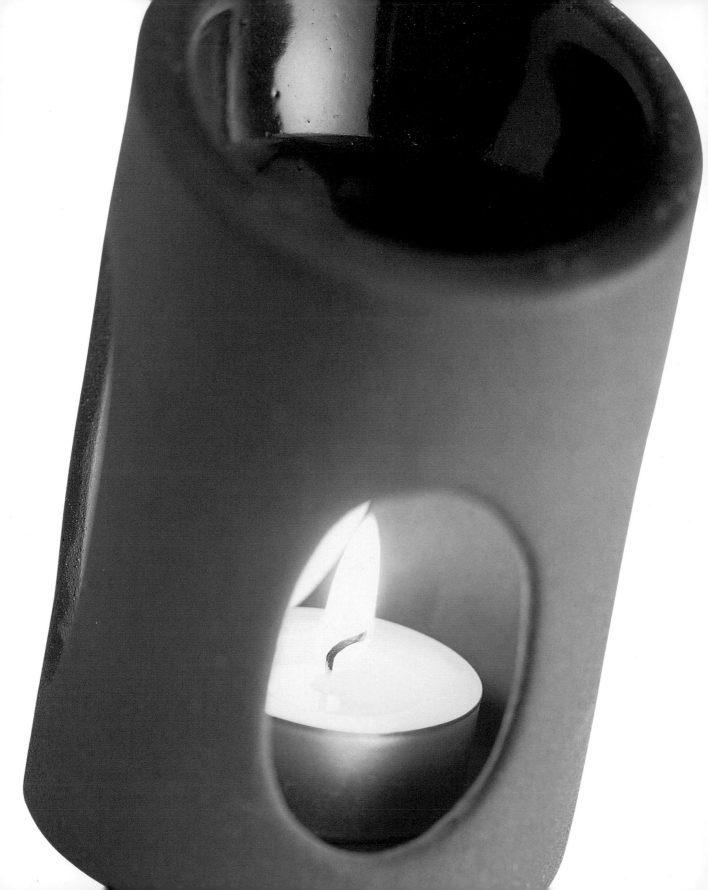

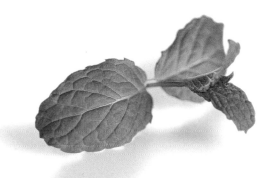

aroma remedies

chrissy wildwood

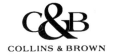

COLLINS & BROWN

IMPORTANT NOTICE

The author and publisher cannot be held responsible for misadventure resulting from the misuse of essential oils, or any other therapeutic method mentioned in this book. Where there is doubt about how to use essential oils, or if there is concern regarding the suitability of home treatment for a particular ailment, do seek the advice of a professional aromatherapist. Should symptoms persist despite sensible use of essential oils, it is important to seek medical advice and to mention that aromatherapy has been used.

First published in Great Britain in 2000
by Collins & Brown Limited
London House
Great Eastern Wharf
Parkgate Road
London SW11 4NQ

Distributed in the United States and Canada by Sterling Publishing Co,
387 Park Avenue South, New York, NY 10016, USA

1 3 5 7 9 8 6 4 2

British Library Cataloguing-in-Publication Data:
A catalogue record for this book
is available from the British Library.

ISBN 1 85585 742 1

Editor: Emma Baxter
Designer: Claire Graham
Photography: Sian Irvine

Reproduction by Global Colour Ltd, Malaysia
Printed and bound in Hong Kong by Dai Nippon Printing Co. Ltd

Contents

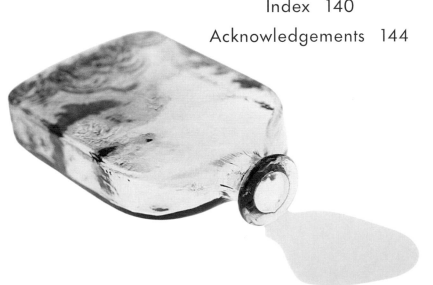

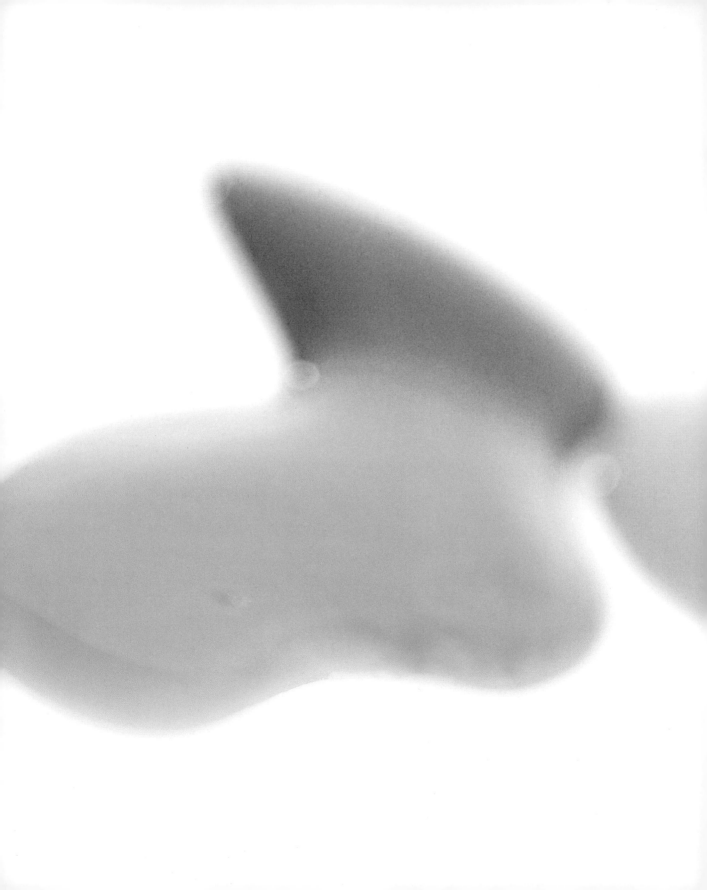

Introduction

The current burgeoning of interest in the practice of aromatherapy, herbalism and other natural methods of healing is part of the movement towards a 'greener' way of living. Instinctively, we are turning to the wonderful healing power of nature to restore a sense of harmony to body and soul.

In common with all natural therapies, aromatherapy is more effective when incorporated as part of a holistic healing plan. This entails looking beyond symptoms to the possible causes and prevention of illness. It is important to remember that ailments do not strike 'out of the blue', even though it may seem that way at times.

There are many possible causes of ill health: heredity plays a part but, in the main, its origin lies in our mental state, lifestyle and diet.

As you will see from the self-help treatments outlined in this book, holistic aromatherapy demands a great deal of commitment. It may not be as easy as merely surrendering your body to a doctor and taking medicine, nor can you expect an overnight cure. However, the long-term benefits – increased vitality and enhanced quality of life – are well worth the effort.

Aromatherapy has many, many virtues, but perhaps the most important is its use as a treatment for dissipating the adverse effects of stress (or distress) in its many guises. There is no longer any medical dispute that emotional distress (including damaging beliefs and strong, unexpressed emotions) can manifest as physical symptoms which then contribute to an overall weakening of the immune system. The aim of holistic treatment is to address the interrelated aspects of our being as a whole: mind, body and spirit (also known as the mind/body complex). Whatever affects one aspect of the self – the body, mind or spirit – affects the whole.

The aim of this book is to provide a concise, yet comprehensive and practical guide to the safe use of essential oils for healing purposes. Even if you know next to nothing about aromatherapy, using this beautifully illustrated manual you will soon confidently be creating your own aroma remedies for the health and emotional well-being of yourself, your family and your friends. Here's wishing you health and contentment.

Chrissy Wildwood

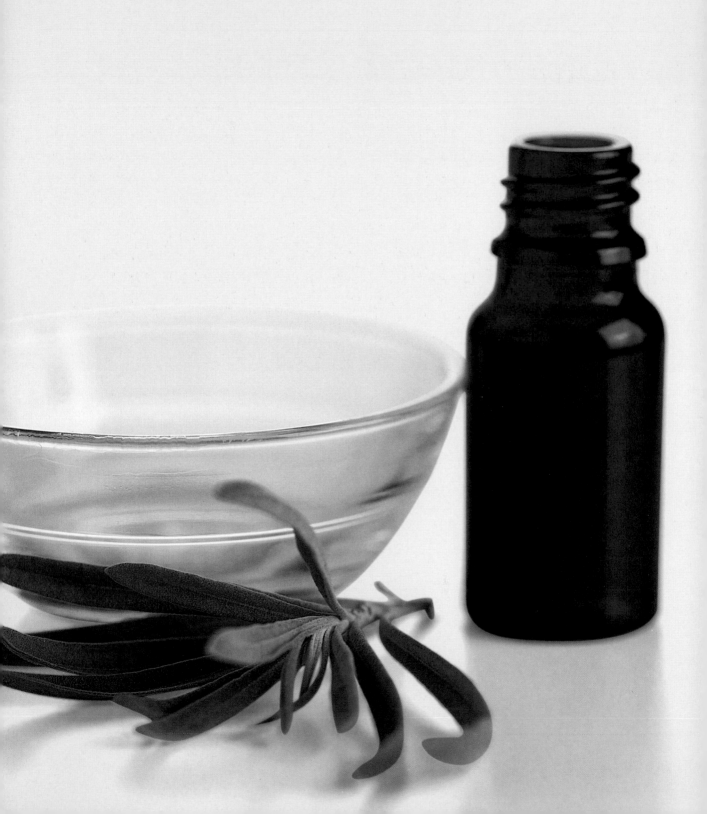

Aromatherapy Foundations

Aromatherapy is the therapeutic use of essential oils. Treatment involves applying these aromatic oils to the body, or simply inhaling them, to improve health and promote a sense of well-being. But what exactly are essential oils, and how do they exert their beneficial effects?

The Nature of Essential Oils

Essential oils, or 'essences' as they are also called, occur naturally in a variety of aromatic plants and trees. They may be found, for example, in flowers (rose, ylang-ylang), leaves (eucalyptus, peppermint), wood (sandalwood, cedarwood), gum resin (frankincense, myrrh), seeds (cardamom, fennel) and citrus rind (lemon).

Even though they are technically classified as 'oils', they are quite different from 'fixed' cooking oils such as sunflower and olive. Essential oils are volatile: they evaporate when left in the open air. Many have the consistency of alcohol, though others, such as myrrh and vetiver, are viscous. While most essences are pale yellow or virtually colourless, others may be greenish (bergamot), amber (patchouli), reddish (carrot seed) or deep blue (German chamomile).

Capturing the Essence

The majority of essential oils are captured by steam distillation, a technique whose origins can be traced to ancient Mesopotamia. Put simply, distillation involves putting the plant material in a large vat and forcing steam through it. The heat and pressure release droplets of essential oil which are carried with the steam. This aromatic vapour moves along a series of glass tubes surrounded by a cold water 'jacket', thus causing it to cool and condense (change back into liquid). The essential oil is then separated from the water by siphoning it off through a narrow-necked container called a florentine.

The oils of citrus fruits are usually extracted by cold expression. This was formerly carried out by squeezing the rind and collecting the oil (the zest) in a sponge, but today, however, machines using the principle of centrifugal force are used.

Fragrance materials can also be extracted using solvents such as hexane and petroleum ether. The resulting product, called an absolute, is not a pure essential oil, as it contains additional plant constituents and traces of residue from the solvent. Absolutes are primarily employed by the perfume industry. Even though some aromatherapists do use absolutes in their treatments, others (including myself) believe the use of these in the extraction process runs counter to the philosophy of aromatherapy, which prides itself on being completely 'natural'. Therefore, such aromatics do not feature in the recipes given in this book.

Properties of Essential Oils

Each oil comprises a unique combination of biochemical components which have different therapeutic properties. Esters, for example, which are found in high quantities in such oils as chamomile and lavender, are excellent anti-inflammatory, antifungal and wound-healing agents and have a soothing effect on the mind. Phenols, found in high concentration in oils such as clove and sage, have a strong antibiotic action and are mentally stimulating. Nevertheless, it is important to remember that essential oils are incredibly complex substances – so complex that it is impossible to isolate their numerous trace elements and compounds. Different essential oils, therefore, have numerous overlapping properties, and it is likely they have other beneficial actions which are as yet unrecognized by science. So a single essential oil can often be helpful for an amazingly broad spectrum of conditions (see Directory of Essential Oils, page 110).

When used in aromatherapy treatments – for example, diluted in a vegetable oil and massaged into the skin or added to bath water – essential oils are absorbed by the body in two different ways: through the skin and by inhalation. The tiny aromatic molecules of an essential oil pass through the hair follicles and into the bloodstream or are taken up by the lymph and interstitial fluid (a liquid surrounding all body cells). Once

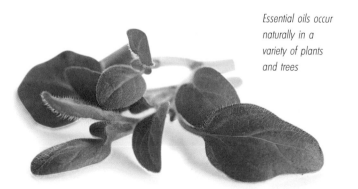

Essential oils occur naturally in a variety of plants and trees

breathed in, they arrive in the lungs from where they diffuse across the tiny air sacs into the surrounding blood capillaries. Having reached the bloodstream, an essential oil may have a pharmacological effect upon the body, even though the amount absorbed is very small.

At the same time, there is the emotional and psychological benefits of aromatherapy. On breathing in the aroma, the essential oil molecules connect with the olfactory receptors in the roof of the nose. These are linked to the limbic system, an area of the brain associated with our instinctive drives: emotion, intuition, memory, creativity, sleep patterns, sex drive and so on. If the aroma is liked, the brain releases neurotransmitters that either relax or stimulate the nervous system. From this, it may be easier to understand how aromatherapy can have a profound effect on our physical and emotional well-being.

◦ Quality Control

Essential oils can vary enormously in price and quality, depending on two main factors: the amount of oil found in the plant material and the integrity of the distillation process. The more oil glands present in the plant, the cheaper the oil, and vice versa. 100 kilos of lavender, for instance, yields almost three litres of essential oil, whereas 100 kilos of rose petals surrenders merely half a litre. A poorly distilled oil may smell 'burnt' or 'stewed' as a result of human error (some plants require a shorter or longer distillation time than average). Poorly distilled oils are unreliable as therapeutic agents, their chemistry may be quite different from oils extracted under optimum conditions, so their effects will vary accordingly.

The quality of aroma is also influenced by the vagaries of climate, geographical location, soil condition, altitude, air quality and probably many other subtle and interrelated factors as yet unrecognized by science. So the aroma of a genuine essential oil will vary from one harvest to the next, just like the bouquet of a good wine. This also explains why the same named oil is likely to smell somewhat different from one supplier to the next.

The majority of essential oils produced are used as food flavouring agents and perfume materials. They are also of some interest to the pharmaceutical industry, but usually only in order for chemists to isolate their 'active principles'. Some, of course, continue to be employed in their natural state by aromatherapists and medical herbalists.

Unfortunately, the demand for essential oils (especially lavender, rose, neroli, geranium and sandalwood) often exceeds world supply. This means that many oils available from high street stores may have been altered or extended in the laboratory to make up for the shortfall, or perhaps adulterated solely to increase profits. They may contain synthetic additives and dilutants, or perhaps isolated components extracted from less expensive essential oils with a similar aroma. Quite apart from problems of decreased potency, such oils pose a greater risk of causing adverse skin reactions and should never be used for aromatherapy.

◖ Where to Buy Essential Oils

Aromatherapists usually purchase essential oils from specialist mail order suppliers, and most firms respond quickly. Since many are also happy to sell small quantities to unqualified essential oil enthusiasts, it's always worth asking an aromatherapist in your area to recommend a supplier. You could also try telephoning an aromatherapy training school to find out which oils they recommend: they may even distribute their own. Good quality oils are also available from certain health food shops, pharmacies and shops specializing in herbs and other natural remedies, but again, it's worth seeking the recommendation of a local aromatherapist.

◖ Always Read the Label

Top quality essential oils should be labelled 'pure and natural', which ought to indicate that they are unblended and contain no synthetic substances. Since the common names for plants and their essential oils vary from one country to another, the botanical name should also be included on the label. For example, not just 'Lavender', but also *Lavandula angustifolia*.

You may also come across a bottle labelled 'Aromatherapy Oil', which usually means it is a mixture of about 2–3 per cent essential oil placed in a carrier such as sweet almond oil, often with vitamin E as a preservative.

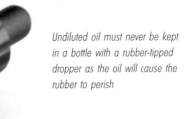

Undiluted oil must never be kept in a bottle with a rubber-tipped dropper as the oil will cause the rubber to perish

GENERAL ESSENTIAL OIL PRECAUTIONS

◆ Keep bottles out of the reach of children.

◆ Generally do not apply neat oils to the skin. One exception is the occasional use of neat lavender or tea tree oil on minor burns and cuts, for example.

◆ Never take essential oils by mouth, vagina (pessary or douche) or rectum (suppository), unless under medical instruction.

◆ Keep essential oils away from the eyes, and do not rub your eyes after handling them. Should any get into the eyes, rinse with plenty of cool water. French aromatherapy practitioners recommend bathing the affected eye with vegetable oil in an eyebath. Essential oils are completely soluble in vegetable oil, but only partially soluble in water, so vegetable oil is certainly the most effective method when a lot of essential oil has splashed into the eyes.

◆ Citrus oils, especially bergamot, increase the skin's sensitivity to ultraviolet light, so do not use on the skin shortly before exposure to sunlight (or a sunbed) as they may cause unsightly pigmentation and increase the risk of sunburn.

◆ Never use an essential oil about which you can find little or no information.

◆ Avoid prolonged use of the same essential oil (i.e. daily for more than two months) as there is a risk of developing a sensitivity to the oil. Take a two-month break before using it again.

◆ If you have sensitive skin, it is advisable to carry out a patch test before using an essential oil for the first time.

◆ If you suffer from asthma, allergic rhinitis or chronic eczema (or have a family history of any of these complaints), home aromatherapy is not recommended. Even professional aromatherapy treatment may not be suitable for all sufferers. Seek the advice of an holistic nutritionist, medical herbalist or homoeopathic practitioner.

◆ If you suffer from asthma, avoid steam inhalations. With or without essential oils, concentrated steam could possibly trigger an attack.

◆ Skin applications of certain essential oils are best avoided during pregnancy. Refer to the CAUTION notes given in the essential oil profiles in the Directory of Essential Oils. Nevertheless, such oils are safe to use in a vaporizer if the aroma is liked.

◆ If you suffer from epilepsy, it is advisable to avoid the essential oils of rosemary, fennel, hyssop and sage, as there is a remote chance that these essences may trigger an attack. Although in certain sufferers any strong odour has the potential to cause a seizure.

◆ Some homoeopaths believe that all essential oils (and other strong odours) can weaken or even cancel out the effects of homoeopathic remedies. Other practitioners believe that only peppermint and eucalyptus should be avoided. Always tell your homoeopath that you are using essential oils.

Always keep bottles away from children

These are fine as ready-mixed massage oils, although an expensive way to enjoy aromatherapy. For instance, a 10ml bottle (the average size) of a diluted essential oil is barely enough for a couple of face and neck massages, whereas 10ml of pure essential oil, once correctly diluted, is enough for countless full-body massages.

Another drawback is that ready-mixed oils are not concentrated enough to be used by the drop to perfume bath water – nor indeed, to use in a burner for fragrancing a room. True, one or two oils like rose otto and neroli are very expensive, so buying the ready-diluted versions can indeed be a good way to begin experimenting with them. But remember, a little bottle of pure oil goes a very long way, so it's always worth the investment!

◦ A Word about Organic Oils

Organic oils are increasingly available from health stores and specialist aromatherapy suppliers, but they are more expensive than those extracted from plants that have been exposed to chemical fertilizers and toxic sprays. When buying citrus oils, however, it is essential to buy an organic product. Citrus fruits are the most heavily sprayed of all crops and therefore appreciable quantities of agrochemicals end up in their essential oils. When buying organic oils always check the label for a recognized name and symbol declaring organic authenticity, such as the Soil Association (UK), Ecocert (France) or Demeter (Germany).

◦ Caring for your Oils

Essential oils evaporate readily and are easily damaged by light, extremes of temperature and exposure to oxygen in the air. For this reason they are sold in well-stoppered, dark glass bottles. The bottle should be equipped with an accurate integral dropper cap. A poorly designed dropper allows the oil to pour out, making it impossible to measure the amount accurately. Rubber-tipped droppers should never be used for essential oils, as the oil will cause the rubber to perish.

In ideal conditions, most essential oils will keep for several years, although the average shelf life is about two years. Most expressed (cold-pressed) citrus oils deteriorate within six to 12 months. All essential oils, however, are vulnerable when exposed to air, particulary pine oils. The more often you open the bottle, the greater the chance of oxidation – a process whereby the oil is chemically combined with oxygen and its original structure altered or destroyed. This change is reflected in the deterioration of aroma. As well as the problem of decreased potency, an oxidized oil is more likely to cause skin irritation.

To prolong the life of your oils, store them in a cool, dry, dark place. Essential oils can also be stored in a refrigerator (enclosed in an airtight food container), although not in the freezer compartment. Citrus oils

Always ensure you buy organic citrus oils

will turn cloudy if stored in cold conditions, but regain their clarity at room temperature.

◦ Shelf Life of Massage Oil Blends

Although neat essential oils have a long shelf life, once diluted in a carrier oil their potency begins to diminish after a few weeks, or even sooner

QUANTITIES AND APPLICATIONS

MASSAGE OIL

Quantity: Adults: 7–15 drops (1.5–3%) in 25ml (1fl. oz.) of carrier oil. Children over 5 years: 2–7 drops (0.5 1.5%) in 25ml (1fl. oz.) of carrier oil.

Further advice: For babies and younger children, please seek professional advice.

OINTMENTS AND CREAMS

Quantity: 10–20 drops in 30g (1oz.) unperfumed ointment or cream base.

Further advice: For bruises, sprains and painful joints, use the maximum concentration of essential oil.

COMPRESS

Quantity: 3–5 drops in 600ml (1pt) hot or cold water.

Further advice: Add oils to bowl of water. Place a cloth on water and wring out. Apply to affected area for five minutes (unless otherwise directed in the recipe section). Repeat 2–4 times. Hot compresses are for dull aches and cramping pain, boils and abcesses. Cold compresses are for recent injuries which feel hot and/or where there is swelling, such as a sprained ankle or wrist.

STEAM INHALATION

Quantity: 2–4 drops in a bowl of very hot water (about 3pts).

Further advice: Add essential oil to bowl of water. Cover bowl and head with a towel to form a 'tent' and inhale for 1–3 minutes. Repeat 2–3 times a day. Effective for respiratory ailments such as bronchitis, coughs, colds and flu. May also be used as a deep-cleansing facial treatment, once or twice weekly.

CAUTION: THIS METHOD MUST BE AVOIDED BY ASTHMA SUFFERERS, AS CONCENTRATED STEAM MY TRIGGER AN ATTACK. WHEN USED AS A FACIAL STEAM TREATMENT, AVOID IF YOU HAVE THREAD VEINS AS HUMIDITY EXACERBATES THE CONDITION.

DRY INHALATION

Quantity: 1–4 drops on a tissue or cotton handkerchief.

Further advice: Inhale at intervals as required. Helpful for colds and flu, to help clear a stuffy head, and for aromatic mood-enhancement.

BATH

Quantity: 4–8 drops (adults) 3–5 drops (10–13 yrs) 2–4 drops (7–9 yrs) 2–3 drops (5–6 yrs)

Further advice: For babies and children under five years, please seek professional advice.

VAPORIZATION

Quantity: For candle-heated vaporizers or 'burners', add 6–15 drops to the water-filled reservoir. For electric vaporizers, follow the manufacturer's instructions.

Further advice: Low quantities are best for aromatic mood-enhancement. Use the maximum concentration as a fumigant when infectious illness is around.

unless stored in a refrigerator. Shop-bought aromatherapy massage oils are usually preserved with vitamin E which has excellent antioxidant properties. Aromatherapists sometimes add the contents of two vitamin E capsules to every 30ml of aromatherapy massage oil. If the blend is stored in a refrigerator (or perhaps a cool, dark cupboard), the shelf life is extended to about three months.

◊ Essential Oil Safety

Essential oils are marvellous healing substances, but they are also highly concentrated and can be potentially hazardous if misused. So, before you begin to experiment, please read the safety guidelines given here.

◊ Carry Out a Patch Test

If you are trying an essential or carrier oil for the first time, it is advisable to conduct a patch test before using it therapeutically. This is particularly important if you have sensitive skin, or want to use the oil on a child. Apply a drop of the oil to the supersensitive spots in the crease of the elbow, behind the ear or on the inside of the wrist. Leave uncovered and unwashed for 24 hours. If there is no redness or itching, the oil is safe to use.

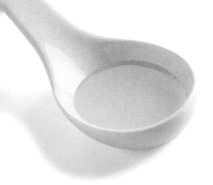

It is very important to measure the correct amount of essential oil

AROMATHERAPY TECHNIQUES

◊ Preparing Essential Oils for Aromatherapy

Although many recipes are given in subsequent chapters, it can be helpful to have some guidance on standard quantities and basic procedures. The chart opposite gives the safest and most commonly used methods for home use. They involve the skin absorption of essential oils through massage, compresses, ointments and baths, as well as inhalation.

For massage, the oils are diluted in a vegetable carrier or base oil such as almond, sunflower, safflower or hazelnut. Try to obtain cold-pressed or unrefined base oils as these contain essential fatty acids and other nutrients which are often destroyed during the refining process. Whenever possible, opt for certified organic essential oils and vegetable oils, produced without the use of poisonous sprays and chemical fertilizers.

AROMATHERAPY SKIN CARE

You may be surprised to learn that it is not advisable to apply an aromatherapy skin-care preparation to your skin every day. Best results are achieved by doing it the French way – by applying correctly diluted essential oils as a periodic 'cure'. This prevents the skin from becoming overly accustomed to the oils and failing to respond positively to them. It also safeguards against the possibility of developing a sensitivity to an aromatherapy formula, which may occur if the same oils are applied daily for months on end. In between times, of course, you may wish to use other natural skin-care products such as those available from health stores and herbal suppliers.

How to Cycle the Treatment

First choose an essential oil (or blend) suitable for your skin type (see the chart on page 18). There are two alternative cycles you could adopt:

Option 1

Apply the oils twice a day for two days a week.

Option 2

Apply the oils once or twice a day for two weeks, then take a four-week interval before resuming with the oils.

Taking the Cure

The most popular methods of application are given below. Experiment to discover which treatment strategy works best for you. You may combine more than one method if desired, but do not exceed the recommended frequency of use during each periodic cure. It should go without saying that the aromatic treatment must be applied to freshly cleansed skin. For your face and neck, use a pH balanced cleansing bar, rather than soap, as this will leave your skin soft and dewy. Soap is alkaline in its action and can leave the more delicate facial skin feeling taut and dry.

• Apply a fine film of your chosen aromatherapy blend immediately after a bath or shower when your skin is still moist with open pores and therefore more receptive to whatever is applied to it.

• Apply 30 minutes after a facial steam or face pack (see Weekly Facials below). Don't apply immediately after these treat-ments as the skin will still be throwing off tissue wastes, a process which hinders absorption.

• Immediately afterwards apply a five-minute warm facial compress. Pour about a pint (600 ml) of comfortably hot water into a heatproof bowl, then immerse two spotlessly clean face flannels in the bowl. Wring out the excess and cover your face (avoiding nostrils and eyes) with the flannels. The easiest way to keep the flannels in place is to lie down on a comfortable surface. You may also wish to put on some tranquil music to help relax your facial muscles.

• Apply shortly before going for a walk or run in the open air, preferably in the park, countryside or along the seashore. The combination of essential oils and fresh air (especially at the seaside or in the mountains) is a marvellous skin rejuvenator.

Weekly Facials

Steam Treatment

Most skins benefit from the deep-cleansing effect of a weekly steam facial, especially oily skin prone to blackheads and spots. However, avoid steaming your skin if you have thread veins as humidity tends to exacerbate the condition. Asthma sufferers should also avoid this type of facial as concentrated steam may trigger an attack.

To carry out a steam facial, fill a heatproof bowl with about a pint (600ml) of near-boiling water.

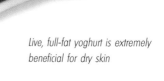

Live, full-fat yoghurt is extremely beneficial for dry skin

To trap the steam, cover your head and the bowl with a towel to form a 'tent'. Stay there for about five minutes (no longer), before splashing you face with tepid water to remove wastes accumulated on the skin's surface. This treatment may be followed by a face pack if you wish.

Face Packs

A weekly face pack deep-cleanses the pores and brightens your complexion by sloughing off dead skin cells.

Two of the finest ingredients for face packs are honey and yoghurt. The yoghurt should be live, full-fat (especially if you have dry skin) and preferably organic. Unless you are allergic to either of these foods, both are beneficial for all skin types. Honey is a marvellous humectant, drawing moisture from the air and imparting a soft dewy glow to skin. The lactic acid in yoghurt helps clear any spots and improves skin tone.

Use either honey or yoghurt, or an equal amount of each mixed together. You will need two to three teaspoons in all. Apply liberally to your face and neck. Leave on for ten to fifteen minutes, then rinse off with tepid water. If using honey (either alone or with yoghurt), apply before stepping into a steamy bath as this boosts its moisturizing properties.

◊ Let Your Skin Breathe

Although the beauty industry encourages us to smother our skins

Eat foods rich in vitamin C
to maintain a healthy glow

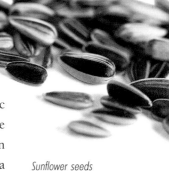

with expensive 'anti-ageing' potions and rich night creams, few people realize that skin needs space to 'breathe'. Prolonged use of chemical-laden cosmetic products interferes with the skin's ability to balance its own secretions and can result in a state of 'product dependency' – which is a condition whereby

Sunflower seeds
are a good source
of vitamin E

the skin feels taut and raw without its daily fix of moisturizer. To encourage your skin to find its own natural balance, provide for breaks in your skin-care routine. For instance, try sleeping product-free at least three times each week. Within a month you should notice a marked improvement in your skin's ability to maintain its own moisture levels.

NUTRITIONAL SUPPORT

As well as following a healthy diet as advocated in the therapeutic sections of this book, the most important vitamins for healthy skin are A, C and E. Eat foods rich in the antioxidant beta-carotene, found in brightly coloured vegetables and fruits, as this is converted by the body into vitamin A. The best sources of vitamin C are citrus fruits and fresh vegetables. Vitamin E, which is added to many skin-care products, can help rehydrate dry skin. Good sources of vitamin E are wheatgerm (found naturally in wholemeal bread), sunflower seeds,

AROMATHERAPY SKINCARE CHART

SKIN TYPE	ESSENTIAL OILS
Normal: soft, smooth and finely textured. Few problems such as spots and flakiness.	Lavender, rose otto, neroli, Roman chamomile, frankincense.
Oily: shiny appearance, usually large pores, prone to blackheads and spots (see also Acne, page 38)	Lavender, German chamomile, rosemary, frankincense, geranium, cypress, juniper berry, Atlas cedarwood, tea tree, carrot seed, myrtle, myrrh.
Combination: the chin, nose and forehead form an oily T-zone on the face, whereas the skin around the eyes, cheeks and neck is dry.	Chamomile (German or Roman), geranium, rose otto, lavender, frankincense, sandalwood.
Dry: feels tight after washing with soap. May also flake and is predisposed to developing facial lines (see also treatment for dry and flaky skin, page 40).	Chamomile (Roman or German), lavender, neroli, rose otto, sandalwood.
Mature: in need of toning and nourishing.	Frankincense, spikenard, carrot seed, rose otto, neroli, sandalwood.
Sensitive: can be of any type, and may become sensitive (inflamed and itchy) from exposure to harsh soaps, cosmetic materials and certain essential oils. Carry out a 24-hour patch test before using any product.	None, unless under the guidance of a qualified aromatherapist. Instead, try infused calendula oil (see page 113) or an unperfumed skin-care product.

RECOMMENDED BASE PRODUCTS

Vegetable oils such as sweet almond, extra virgin olive (mixed up to 50:50 with a lighter base oil), jojoba, safflower, sunflower seed, hazelnut. Lotion or light cream.

SUGGESTED RECIPE

20ml jojoba
1 drop frankincense
1 drop lavender
1 drop neroli
Add essential oils to jojoba and mix well.

Aloe vera gel, light lotion.

25ml aloe vera gel
1 drop myrtle
1 drop rosemary
1 drop lavender
Add oils to gel and stir well.

Light base oils such as jojoba, sweet almond, hazelnut, rosehip seed and infused calendula. Aloe vera gel mixed up to 50:50 with unperfumed lotion.

15ml unperfumed lotion
10ml aloe vera gel
1 drop frankincense
1 drop geranium
1 drop sandalwood
1 drop lavender
Mix together lotion and gel, then stir in oils.

Vegetable oils such as avocado, evening primrose, extra virgin olive (mixed 50:50 with a lighter oil like sweet almond), safflower, sunflower seed. Rich skin cream.

15g rich skin cream
5ml avocado oil
2 drops Roman chamomile
3 drops rose otto
1 drop sandalwood
Stir avocado oil into cream, add oils and mix.

Vegetable oils such as avocado, sweet almond, evening primrose, jojoba, safflower, sunflower seed. Rich skin cream or lotion.

20g unperfumed skin cream
Contents 2 x 500mg evening primrose oil capsules
1 drop carrot seed
Pierce oil capsules with pin and squeeze contents into cream. Add essential oils and mix well.

Infused calendula oil, aloe vera gel. Unperfumed cream or lotion.

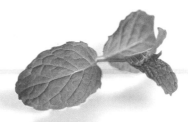

almonds and eggs. One of the finest nutritional supplements is evening primrose oil which contains a high level of gamma linolenic acid (GLA), an essential fatty acid which has been found to increase the moisture level of skin cells.

AROMATHERAPY SKINCARE CHART

Choose between one and three oils from the list of essences recommended for your particular skin type, then mix with a suitable base product. For face and neck treatments, there is usually no need to exceed a one per cent dilution (one drop of essential oil to one teaspoon of vegetable oil, cream or lotion). If using aloe vera gel as a base, as little as 0.5 per cent dilution (one drop of essential oil to two teaspoons of gel) is usually enough. (See page 18 for chart.)

ADDITIONAL TECHNIQUES FOR HOME USE

Body massage is the mainstay of professional aromatherapy, but it cannot be learned from a book. If you would like to master the art of massage, it is essential to enrol on a course of instruction (see Useful Addresses, page 138).

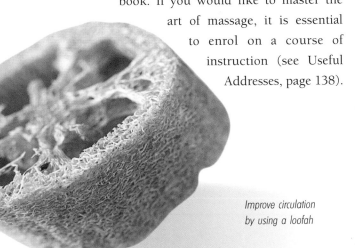

Improve circulation by using a loofah

However, you can derive a great deal of benefit from two self-help procedures: dry skin brushing and self-massage. As well as enhancing the effects of aromatherapy treatments, these quick and simple techniques for use in the home can also be a marvellous addition to your daily health care routine.

● Dry Skin Brushing

Dry skin brushing is excellent for stimulating lymphatic drainage (see page 65) and assisting the elimination of body wastes. It also greatly improves the clarity and texture of the skin by sloughing off dead skin cells which accumulate on the surface. Many health experts believe that skin brushing is similar in body stimulation terms to a professional full-body massage. You will need a purpose-designed vegetable bristle brush with a long, but detachable handle so that you can reach your back (these are easily available from good health stores). If you are unable to obtain a body brush, a hemp glove or loofah will suffice.

The body needs to be brushed once a day – or at least three times a week – for a few minutes before your morning bath or shower. To brush your skin, make sweeping movements over each part of your body. Be gentle: brush too vigorously, especially if you are unused to body brushing, and you will scratch your skin. Begin with your feet, including the soles, then move up your legs, front and back. Brush over the buttocks and up to the middle of your back – that is, always sweeping towards the heart. Then brush your hands, front and back, up the arms, across the shoulders and down the chest (being very careful to avoid the nipples). Finally, brush the abdomen (avoiding the genitals) using a clockwise circular motion following the shape of the colon.

CAUTION: Skin-brushing should be avoided where there is eczema, psoriasis or any other type of skin complaint. Avoid brushing over varicose veins.

◌ Self-Massage

A good time to give yourself a massage is immediately after a warm bath or shower as the oils will penetrate the skin more readily when it is damp and the pores are open. Your strokes should always be towards the heart to improve the circulation. Warm a little oil by rubbing it in your hands, then starting with your feet and legs, stroke the skin hand-over-hand in an upwards direction. Obviously, you will need to massage each arm using the flat of the other hand. Begin with light strokes and gradually let them become firmer.

Once you have stimulated the circulation by stroking, knead the fleshy areas such as thighs, calves and buttocks, it will be easier if you do this while sitting on a towel on the floor (or in the empty bath), with your knees bent slightly and your feet flat on the surface. This will loosen the leg muscles sufficiently to make kneading easier and more comfortable. The massage stroke is similar to kneading bread, it comprises alternately squeezing and releasing handfuls of flesh in a broad circular motion to relax tense muscles.

To massage your abdomen, either stand, or lie on your back. Gently circle the area in a clockwise direction, using the flat of your hand, to aid digestion. Finish the massage the way you began with the hand-over-hand stroking.

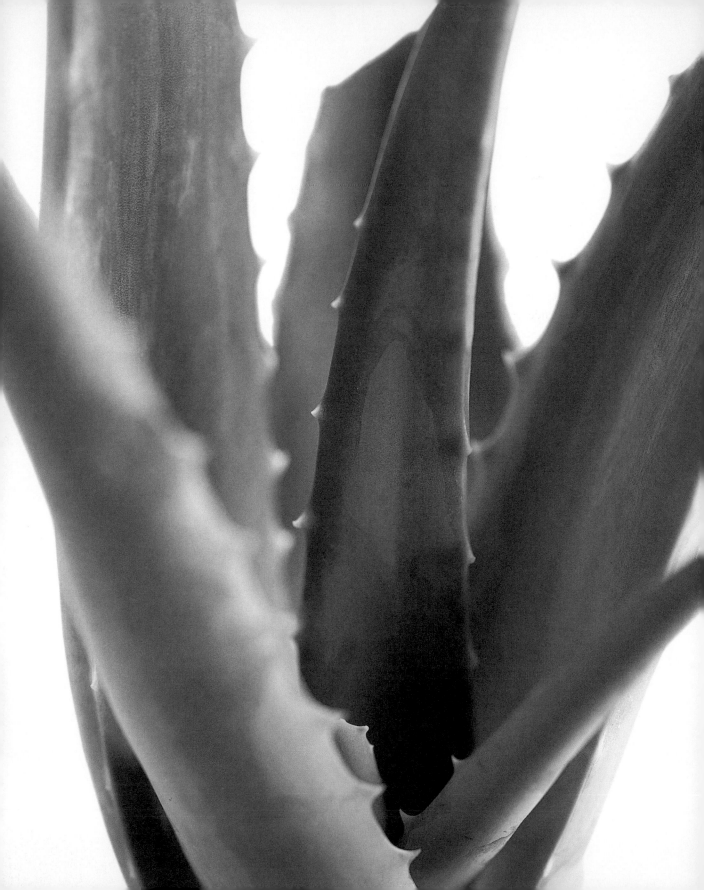

Aromatherapy Store Cupboard

With such a vast array of essential oils from which to choose, you may be wondering where to begin! You could get by on just two essences: lavender and tea tree. If you intend to take the art of aromatherapy seriously, however, you will need a basic starter selection of ten carefully chosen oils, enough to create a variety of fragrant compositions for many common ailments. You may wish to start with the first five oils listed, as these generally are regarded as the most useful, and add to these gradually as you become more familiar with their qualities and uses.

Aromatherapy Starter Kit

Essential Oils: Lavender, tea tree, Roman chamomile, rosemary, geranium, lemon, clary sage, juniper berry, frankincense, ylang-ylang.

Carrier Oil: Sweet Almond

Essential Oil Vaporizer: A candle-heated (or electric) device used to disperse essential oils throughout the atmosphere. Vaporizers are often used for mood-enhancement or fumigation and are available from health stores, craft shops and aromatherapy suppliers.

AROMATHERAPY BASE INGREDIENTS

In the recipe sections of this book, essential oils are blended with other natural ingredients with healing properties of their own. Let's take a closer look at these products and their specific uses in aromatherapy.

VEGETABLE OILS, FATS AND WAXES
◆ Olive Oil

The oil is extracted from the hard, unripe fruits of the olive tree (*Olea europaea*) native to the Mediterranean. There are several grades of olive oil, ranging from highly refined versions with a slight odour, through to the heavy-textured, richly odoriferous, 'extra virgin' grade obtained from the first pressing of the olives. For aromatherapy massage, a good choice is virgin olive oil which is obtained from the second pressing of the fruit. Although still heavy-textured, it has a less pungent aroma than the other grades. Both extra virgin and virgin olive oil contain essential fatty acids and vitamin E. To lessen its odour and heavy texture, blend 50:50 with lighter oils such as sunflower or sweet almond. Both refined and unrefined olive oil is available from supermarkets everywhere.

Avocado oil helps soften dry or mature skin

Avocado Oil

The finest quality avocado oil is cold pressed from the flesh of the avocado (*Persea americana*), a fruit which is native to South America. It has a sludgy appearance (indicating that it has not been damaged by heat and excessive refining) and an emerald green hue. Refined avocado oil is a pale yellow colour with very little odour and few nutrients. The cold-pressed oil is rich in essential fatty acids (essential in that they cannot be produced by the body and must be obtained from the diet) beta-carotene and vitamin E. Despite its viscosity, avocado oil has excellent powers of penetration. It makes a superb treatment oil for dry and mature skins. It can also be taken internally in capsule form (available from pharmacies) to prevent skin dryness and dehydration, such as that caused by excessive sunbathing. For external use the oil is available in bottles from specialist aromatherapy suppliers.

Hazelnut Oil

The oil is warm-pressed from hazelnuts, the fruits of a small tree (*Corylus avellana*) native to North America and Europe. The oil contains useful amounts of essential fatty acids, including linolenic acid. Hazelnut oil has a strong, sweet, nutty aroma and an exceptionally fine texture. It is also highly penetrative and has a slightly astringent effect on the skin. Available from good supermarkets, health stores or from specialist aromatherapy suppliers.

Hazelnuts contain essential fatty acids

Safflower Oil

The oil is extracted from the tiny seeds of the safflower (*Carthamus tinctorius*), a thistle-like plant native to India and China. The unrefined oil is rich in the omega-6 group of essential fatty acids, and contains appreciable quantities of vitamin E. It has a rich, golden colour and slightly nutty aroma. However, it is one of the least stable oils and difficult to keep fresh, so must be stored in a refrigerator. The refined version contains fewer nutrients, though has a longer shelf-life.

Grapeseed Oil

As its name suggests the oil is extracted from the seeds of the grape vine (*Vitis vinifera*). The oil is unavailable in its cold-pressed form because it is considered to be unpalatable, having a sludgy appearance and unpleasant odour. The refined oil has an attractive green tint and an exceptionally fine texture. It is also virtually odourless, hence its popularity with aromatherapists who prefer to use bland base oils for body massage. Being a highly refined oil, it contains only traces of fat-soluble nutrients such as vitamin E.

Sunflower Oil

The oil is extracted from the seeds of the giant sunflower (*Helianthus annus*). Most sunflower oil is highly refined and therefore has few nutrients. It has a slight odour and is pale to dark yellow in colour. The unrefined version is labelled 'Sunflower Seed' and has a slightly sweet, nutty odour and a fine texture. It contains essential fatty acids and a high level of vitamin E. Useful as an inexpensive all-purpose carrier for essential oils. Both varieties of sunflower oil are available from supermarkets and health stores.

Sweet Almond Oil

The oil extracted from the kernels of the sweet almond tree (*Prunus amygdalis* var. *dulcis*), is fairly light-textured with a pale yellow hue. Sweet almond oil has a fairly light texture and pale yellow hue. It is the most popular carrier for essential oils. For body massage, it provides good 'slip' over the skin and is not absorbed too quickly. The refined versions of almond oil available from pharmacies are virtually odourless and devoid of nutrients. The unrefined version is usually only available from specialist aromatherapy suppliers. It has a delicate nutty aroma and contains essential fatty acids and vitamin D.

Evening Primrose Oil

The oil is extracted from the tiny seeds of the evening primrose (*Oenothera biennis*), a yellow-flowered plant native to North America. The oil is rich in a type of fatty acid known as gamma-linolenic acid (GLA) which has anti-inflammatory properties and is especially helpful for dry, inflamed or irritated skin. Although sometimes

Evening primrose oil has anti-inflammatory properties

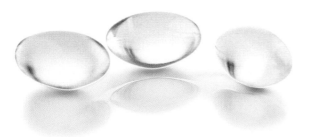

available by the bottle, the oil is exceptionally vulnerable to oxidation (rancidity) upon exposure to air. Far better to buy evening primrose oil capsules and add the contents to home-made skin creams as directed. Available from health stores and pharmacies.

Castor Oil

A thick, sticky oil extracted from the seeds of a small, thorny plant (*Ricinus communis*). It is used in commercial hair conditioners, barrier creams, lipsticks and even eye drops. Castor oil is also particularly useful as an emollient in home-made lip salves. The oil is available from pharmacies and shops specializing in herbal remedies and natural cosmetic materials.

Cocoa Butter

Cocoa butter is obtained by grinding roasted cacao beans and separating the vegetable fat. Women on West Indian cocoa plantations used this chocolate-scented buttery pomade to protect and soften the skin, and prevent stretch marks during pregnancy. It is a popular ingredient in commercial face, body and hand creams, and makes an excellent addition to home-made aromatherapy skin creams. Even though it is a solid, cocoa butter melts at body temperature making it easy to apply. Available from shops specializing in herbal remedies and home-made cosmetic materials.

Beeswax

Bees secrete wax to seal the honeycomb in which they store honey and flower pollen. After the honey is extracted, the combs are placed in hot water and the wax skimmed off and allowed to

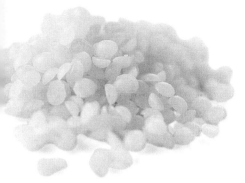

Mix beeswax granules with vegetable oil to create a skin cream

harden. Beeswax is used in many skin creams and lotions. It protects skin against excessive moisture loss, but without clogging the pores. When melted and mixed with vegetable oil, it makes an excellent carrier for essential oils. Available from craft shops and herbal suppliers, either in small blocks, or as easy-to-melt granules.

HERBAL PRODUCTS

◖ Hypercal Ointment

A marvellous skin-healing product containing extracts of St John's wort (*Hypericum perforatum*) and marigold flowers (*Calendula officinalis*). Indispensible to the natural first-aid kit for cuts, minor burns, sores, rashes and abrasions. It may also be combined with appropriate essential oils for treating cold sores and athlete's foot. Available from health stores and pharmacies.

◖ Aloe Vera Gel

Extracted from the succulent African plant, *Aloe barbadensis*. Its plump, tapering leaves exude a thick, clear gel when cut and squeezed. Helpful for inflamed skin conditions such as eczema and minor burns (including sunburn). It also makes an effective moisturizer for oily and congested skin, and may be used as a carrier for essential oils when a non-greasy product is preferred. Available from health stores. When choosing an aloe vera product, check the label to ensure that it contains at least 85 per cent of the plant extract.

◖ Hypericum Tincture

This healing and antiseptic tincture is prepared from the leaves and flowers of St John's wort. It is obtained by macerating the plant material in a mixture of alcohol and water. When taken internally as a herbal medicine (half a teaspoon diluted in a teacupful of water three times daily), research confirms that this remedy works as an anti-depressant and sedative. Applied externally in an ointment or lotion base it soothes and heals burns, cuts, wounds and sores. Often mixed 50:50 with calendula tincture which reinforces its skin-healing properties. Available from herbal suppliers and health stores (see also the Hypericum profile on page 124).

◖ Calendula Tincture

This soothing, healing and antiseptic tincture is prepared from marigold flowers. It is obtained by macerating the flowers in a mixture of alcohol and water. Incorporated into ointments or lotions it soothes and heals sore, cracked or inflamed skin, insect bites and stings, minor burns, scalds, cuts and grazes. It

Calendula flowers are made into a healing tincture

also has fungicidal properties making it an effective treatment for conditions such as athlete's foot and ringworm. It is often mixed 50:50 with hypericum tincture which serves to reinforce its skin-healing properties. Calendula tincture is available from herbal suppliers and health stores (see also the Calendula profile on page 113).

GROCERY ITEMS
Honey

The healing properties of honey have been known for centuries. Applied externally, its antiseptic properties promote the healing of acne-prone skin and sunburn. When added to bath water, incorporated into home-made ointments or used as a face mask, it softens and moisturizes the skin. It also makes a good carrier for essential oils in various therapeutic applications. The best honey is cold-pressed (not pasturized) and slightly cloudy. This indicates that the honey has retained a good concentration of pollen with its complement of vitamins and enzymes. Available from beekeepers, quality grocers and health shops.

Milk

When added to bath water, the lactic acid in milk gently exfoliates the skin and enhances its ability to retain moisture, leaving it silky smooth. Goat's milk is best for skin treatments and even helps relieve certain forms of eczema. It also makes a good facial cleanser suitable for all skin types, and is particularly helpful for oily and blemished complexions.

Oats

Oats are extremely soothing when applied to the skin. In the form of flakes or meal, they can be used as a gentle scrub to slough off dead skin cells, made into a bath bag to soften the skin (this is especially beneficial where there is eczema), or applied as a face pack (mixed with enough spring-water or yoghurt to form a paste) to deep-cleanse and brighten the complexion.

Rice Flour

A fine, cream-coloured flour made from finely ground white rice. It has a lovely silky texture and was a popular face powder until the twentieth century. Sifted until fluffy and sediment-free, rice flour is a healthy alternative to commercial talcum powders which often contain boric acid and synthetic perfume, both of which can irritate sensitive skin. Rice flour is available from good health food shops.

Yoghurt

Fresh, live, full-fat yoghurt (preferably organic and without additional ingredients) is an excellent skin-care agent for all skin types, particularly excessively dry or oily skin. The lactic acid in yoghurt is similar to that of the skin's acid mantle, and appears to balance the secretion of sebum

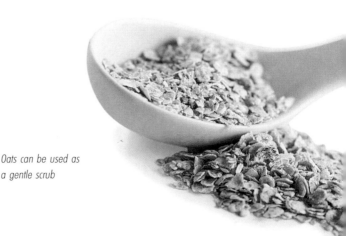

Oats can be used as a gentle scrub

(the skin's own lubricating fluid). It is especially beneficial when applied as a face or body pack (perhaps combined with green clay) for treating oily and congested skin. Available from health stores and supermarkets.

◊ Cider Vinegar

Cider vinegar contains about five per cent malic acid. Most other vinegars, except naturally fermented wine vinegar (popular in France), are too acidic for use on the skin. In skin tonics, hair tonics and friction rubs, it helps to restore the skin's acid/alkaline, or pH, balance, measured on a scale of 0 to 14. Healthy skin registers between 5.4 and 6.2, a mildly acidic condition which acts as a protection against infection. When used as a carrier in water-based aromatherapy lotions, cider vinegar makes essential oils disperse more evenly. Once in contact with the skin, the smell of vinegar wears off within a few seconds. Available from supermarkets and health stores.

◊ Cornflour

Also known as cornstarch, this is made from finely ground maize or sweetcorn kernels. It is useful as a body powder and can be used on its own or with the addition of essential oils (see Rice Flour, page 27). Available from supermarkets and grocers.

MINERAL PRODUCTS
◊ Dead Sea Salts

The salts are collected from the shores of the Dead Sea and have been recognized for their healing properties for more than two thousand years. They contain magnesium, potassium, calcium and trace minerals. Added to bath water the salts relieve aching joints and muscular pain, alleviate dry and flaky skin disorders, and generally relax and revitalize a depleted nervous system. Available from pharmacies and health stores.

◊ Green Clay

The Egyptians, Greeks and Romans all used clay treatments (internally and externally) to detoxify the system, heal wounds, alleviate athletic aches and pains, rejuvenate the skin and promote a sense of well-being. Today, there are several types of clay used for health and beauty treatments, including kaolin (white clay), although green clay is the most popular. Green clay contains a wide range of minerals and trace elements such as silica, magnesium, titanium, iron and calcium. However, it is unsuitable for sensitive and dry skins. Available from health stores, pharmacies and herbal suppliers.

DISTILLED WATERS
◊ Distilled and Purified Water

Distilled water is used in a number of recipes given in this book. Never incorporate ordinary tap water (or even bottled spring water) into skin creams and lotions as it harbours micro-organisms which rapidly multiply and diminish the keeping qualities of such products. Distilled water remains fresh for much longer. Available from pharmacies.

◊ Rosewater

Rosewater has been used for centuries as an ingredient in skin creams and toners. Like orange-flower water, it is often a by-product of

Rose petals used for distillation

the distillation process used to obtain the essential oil. However, because it takes a vast quantity of fresh rose petals to produce a tiny amount of rose oil, some distilleries only make rosewater as this can be produced from a relatively modest weight of flowers. As with other floral waters, the genuine product is available only from specialist aromatherapy suppliers (see Orange Flower Water below). Rosewater makes a pleasant toner or aftershave suitable for all skin types, including dry, sensitive and mature complexions. It may also be used in a vaporizer for its soothing and uplifting effect.

◊ Witch Hazel

Witch hazel (*Hamamelis virginiana*) is a small, twisted, woodland tree native to North America. Native American tribes used decoctions of the bark in poultices for swellings and tumours. The witch hazel commonly available from pharmacies is extracted by steam distillation of the leaves and twigs, with alcohol added as a preservative. It is a well-known first-aid remedy for treating cuts, bruises and swellings.

◊ Orange Flower Water

Orange flower water is a by-product of the distillation process used to obtain the essential oil known as neroli. Most of the orange flower available from high street pharmacies is reconstituted from a synthetic concentrate. The genuine product (collected directly from the still) is known as a 'hydrolat' or 'hydrosol', but is available only from specialist aromatherapy suppliers. A good alternative floral water (available from some essential oil suppliers) is made by dissolving the essential oil of neroli (or rose) in a little alcohol, which is then further diluted in distilled water.

Orange flower water is slightly more astringent than rosewater and makes a good skin tonic or aftershave for oily complexions, and can be incorporated into skin creams in place of distilled water. It may also be used in a vaporizer for its relaxing and uplifting properties.

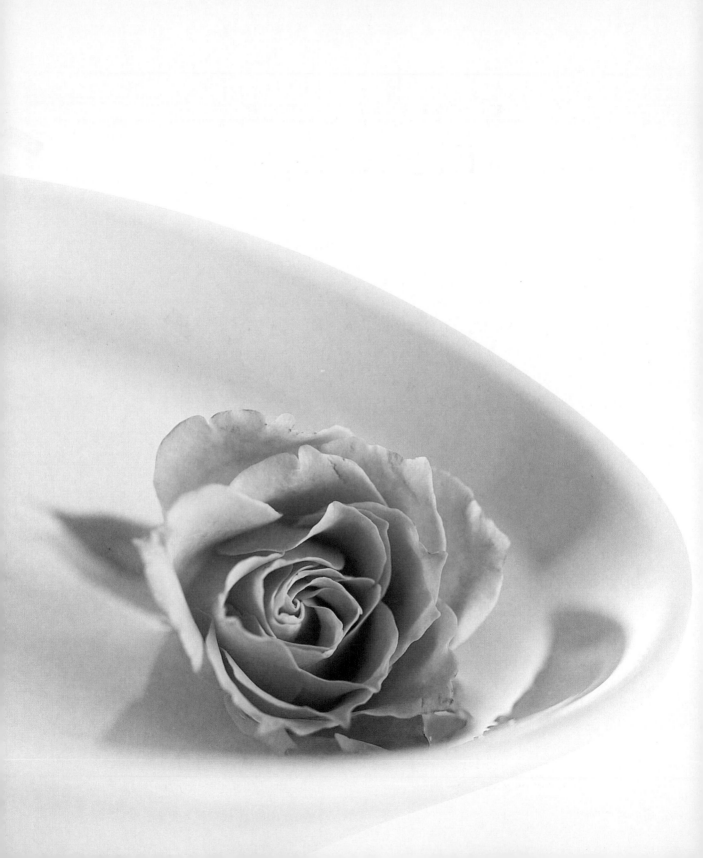

Aromatherapy Blending

Creating aromatic prescriptions and mood-enhancing room scents is immensely enjoyable and therapeutic in itself. Although many recipes are given in this book, here you will learn the basic principles of aromatherapy blending to enable you to develop personalized formulas for yourself, your family and friends.

Aroma Preference

Essential oils may be used singly, although aromatherapists like to blend two, three or more together to match an individual's physical and emotional needs. They also usually smell better when a few are mixed together, and appreciation of the fragrance is an important part of the treatment. While oils such as tea tree and eucalyptus are generally thought of as medicinal-smelling and rose and ylang-ylang as sweet and floral, our perception of pleasant and unpleasant is often highly personal, dependent upon our genetic make-up, personality and our memories which are associated with certain smells.

Studies have shown that pleasurable sensations (incuding the enjoyment of scent) trigger the release of brain hormones such as endorphins and encephalins which are the body's natural opiates or 'happiness' chemicals. The receptors for these substances are found in other parts of the body, such as the skin, and on white blood cells (called

monocytes) in the immune system, their role being to support the body's self-healing processes.

Odour researchers employing EEG (electro-encephalograph) instruments, that record electrical activity in the brain, found that if someone dislikes the aroma of an essential oil – especially if it elicits a gut-felt 'ugh!' – its potentially positive effect on the central nervous system is effectively blocked. So, although some oils are sedative, anti-depressant or stimulating, if the aroma is perceived as unpleasant you are unlikely to respond in the right way to its mood-enhancing properties.

Eucalyptus has a camphor-like aroma

Aromatherapists know that we tend to be instinctively drawn to the essential oil (or blend) which best suits our physical and emotional needs at a given time. For the same reason, we can develop a dislike of certain aromas when we no longer need their properties. For instance, it is common for pre-menstrual women to be attracted to the warm, sweet fragrance of Roman chamomile, a mildly sedative oil which is also helpful for headaches, skin eruptions and insomnia – common symptoms of PMS. Yet the same oil may well be perceived as 'sweet and cloying' when it is no longer needed.

Unlike chemical drugs and synthetic odorants, which are composed of relatively few chemical compounds, nature's essential oils are complex. A single oil may contain hundreds of biochemical components, so all essential oils have multiple properties, many of them shared. This means that if you dislike the aroma of a particular oil, there is likely to be another you can use instead.

Perfume Notes

Some aromatherapists take into account the 'perfume notes' of a blend. According to this system, a well-balanced blend is composed of top notes, middle notes and base notes (the perfume note of each oil is included in the profiles in the Directory of Essential Oils). Top notes (such as citrus oils) are highly volatile so their scent evaporates very quickly. Middle notes (such as rose, neroli and rosemary) last a little longer and impart warmth and fullness to the blend. Base notes (such as patchouli, vetiver and sandalwood) are tenacious or long-lasting, and able to 'fix' other aromas – slowing down the evaporation of top and middle notes to increase the blend's staying power.

However, knowledge of perfume notes is not essential; after all, the system was invented by a perfumer, not an aromatherapist. Take the base notes: none of the oils in this group would be suitable for use in a vaporizer (or inhaled from a tissue) to promote mental alertness. To sharpen the mind, choose highly volatile oils with a piercing or refreshing quality, such as lemon, peppermint, pine or rosemary (top and middle notes). It would be counterproductive to add a heavy base note like sandalwood or vetiver to such a blend, as these oils tend to lull the mind.

Happy Aroma Families

Another way to look at blending is to be guided by the principle that 'families' of aromas generally blend harmoniously. Certain oils have qualities which belong to more than one family, however. The scent of lavender, for example, is both herbaceous and floral in character, while vetiver emanates earth and wood nuances. Aside from such ambiguities, the table below lists five families and examples of harmonious compositions. Other compatible blends are: spices with citrus (such as ginger, lemon and bergamot), florals with citrus (such as ylang-ylang and lemon), peppery notes with woods (such as juniper berry and cedarwood), and resins with floral and citrus (such as frankincense, rose and mandarin). Woods and resins are a good match too: frankincense and cedarwood is a classic. Oils from the aromatic grass family combine well, especially the lemony, floral scent of palmarosa with a hint of lemongrass. Try marrying wildly differing personalities,

HERBACEOUS:
Rosemary, marjoram and peppermint

CITRUS:
Bergamot, mandarin and lemon

FLORAL
Rose, neroli and ylang-ylang

WOODY:
Cedarwood and sandalwood

EARTHY:
Vetiver and patchouli

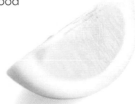

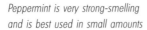

Peppermint is very strong-smelling and is best used in small amounts

such as the ancient and enigmatic frankincense with everyday lavender; rose-scented geranium with a trace (but no more!) of peppermint; or heady neroli with a hint of earthy patchouli or vetiver.

Two good all-rounders are clary sage and petitgrain. Although rather uninteresting and seemingly incomplete when used alone, they blend well with most other oils. Individually (or mixed together), they may be used as a 'bridge' to connect highly volatile oils like bergamot and mandarin with deeply resonating oils like cedarwood and sandalwood.

Making Highly Odoriferous Oils Work in a Blend

Certain essential oils are highly odoriferous, which means they will dominate your blends unless used sparingly. Until your nose has become familiar with the odour intensity of different oils, it is advisable to refer to the 'odour intensity' note included in each of the profiles in the Directory of Essential Oils.

Tea tree is one of the hardest oils to blend. Its strong, medicinal odour tends to overpower most others, although it does work when harmonized with larger amounts of citrus oils, especially lemon. Other highly odoriferous oils are lemongrass, palmarosa, patchouli, cistus, peppermint and vetiver. When experimenting – say, to create a massage blend – add a single drop to 25ml of carrier oil. Add other essential oils drop by drop,

smelling as you go, until you achieve a desirable combination. If using a highly odoriferous oil in the bath, use just a single drop, plus a few drops of a compatible oil.

Preliminary Smell Test

Before you begin mixing your chosen oils, this test will give you a rough idea of the finished formula. First, make some smelling strips by cutting blotting paper into narrow pieces (if you prefer, purpose-designed strips are available from essential oil suppliers). Put a single drop of essential oil on the end of a smelling strip, using a separate strip for each oil. Fashion the papers into a fan-shape, then waft them under your nose to encourage vaporization. Do you like the aroma overall? Experiment for a while, replacing one oil with another. Enjoy discovering how different essential oils smell when you put them together.

Creating a Healing Formula

First select an oil which best matches your symptoms and has an aroma you like. For example, you may be suffering from nervous tension and muscular pain. Lavender would

Smelling strips are easy to make and allow you to experiment with different blends

be an excellent choice (if you like the aroma), perhaps blended with a little frankincense and neroli. If you are not keen on lavender, there are numerous other oils which can relax taut muscles and soothe the mind – for example, cedarwood, clary sage and chamomile. Any of these oils could form the basis of your blend, supported with compatible oils.

To help you choose oils which combine well, refer to the blending advice details included in each of the profiles in the Directory of Essential Oils, though do ensure that you take into account the properties of every oil used in the blend. If, for example, you intend to create a relaxing formula based on rose, you might choose other calming oils such as chamomile, neroli and clary sage. Even though oils such as ginger, black pepper, cardamom and coriander are listed as being compatible with rose, in this instance their stimulating qualities would be counterproductive.

When choosing oils for another person, refine the process of selection (and help guard against olfactory fatigue) by singling out six to eight possibles chosen according to the properties of the oils and the individual's prevalent physical and emotional symptoms. Allow the person to choose between one and four oils according to their preference. If more than one oil is chosen, apply your blending skills to create a well-balanced formula. Remember, the aromatic

Ginger has stimulating properties

prescription may need to be changed from time to time, in accordance with the fluctuating needs of the person you are treating.

Although the art of aromatherapy blending may at first seem daunting, with dedication and enthusiasm you will be surprised how quickly your blending skills develop. It's reassuring to remember that almost any combination of oils is a potentially harmonious blend, provided the oils are mixed in the correct ratio. As there are thousands upon thousands of potentially compatible combinations, begin by taking into account the therapeutic properties of your chosen essential oils, then allow your nose to guide you. Soon you will be creating a cornucopia of aromatic formulas which are both aesthetically pleasing and therapeutic. Your apprenticeship begins right here!

Therapeutic Blending Chart

The information given on the chart opposite demonstrates the basic principles of therapeutic blending, just to get you started. It would take forever to explore every conceivable permutation. So this chart highlights two important therapeutic actions of six popular essential oils and demonstrates how these properties may be enhanced. It also takes into account the aesthetic quality of each blend. As you will see, even 'stimulating' oils like peppermint can be made tranquil if used sparingly with soothing, aroma-compatible oils like lavender and clary sage; while 'relaxing' ylang-ylang becomes invigorating when combined with lemongrass and coriander. (For further information on properties and compatibility see the Directory of Essential Oils, page 110).

THERAPEUTIC BLENDING CHART

ESSENTIAL OIL	PROPERTIES IN FOCUS	BLENDS TO ENHANCE PROPERTIES
Lavender	Sedative, anti-rheumatic	SEDATIVE VAPORIZING BLEND: 3 drops lavender, 1 drop peppermint, 2 drops clary sage. ANTI-RHEUMATIC MASSAGE OIL: 25ml olive oil, 5 drops lavender, 2 drops sweet marjoram, 1 drop ginger, 2 drops lemon.
Rosemary	Mental stimulant, muscle relaxant	MENTALLY STIMULATING DRY INHALATION (drops on tissue): 1 drop rosemary, 1 drop cardomom. MUSCLE RELAXANT MASSAGE OIL: 25ml olive oil, 4 drops rosemary, 2 drops Scots pine, 2 drops Virginian cedarwood, 3 drops lavender.
Sweet marjoram	Expectorant, antiseptic	CHEST RUB FOR CATARRH: 25ml sweet almond oil, 4 drops sweet marjoram, 4 drops Atlas cedarwood, 3 drops eucalyptus. ANTISEPTIC OINTMENT: 20g unperfumed skin cream, 4 drops sweet marjoram, 5 drops lavender, 4 drops tea tree.
Juniper berry	Sedative, diuretic	SEDATIVE BATH BLEND: 1 drop juniper berry, 1 drop sandalwood, 1 drop clary sage, 3 drops mandarin. MASSAGE OIL FOR MINOR FLUID RETENTION (as in PMS): 25ml sweet almond oil, 4 drops juniper berry, 2 drops geranium, 1 drop carrot seed, 3 drops grapefruit.
Rose otto	Antidepressant, anti-inflammatory	ANTI-DEPRESSANT BATH BLEND: 2 drops rose otto, 1 drop lime, 1 drop petitgrain, 1 drop orange, 2 drops bergamot. ANTI-INFLAMMATORY GEL FOR SUNBURN: 35ml aloe vera gel, 1 drop rose otto, 1 drop German chamomile, 1 drop lavender.
Ylang-ylang	Sedative, circulatory stimulant	SEDATIVE MASSAGE OIL: 25ml sweet almond oil, 2 drops ylang-ylang, 2 drops sandalwood, 4 drops mandarin. MASSAGE OIL FOR SLUGGISH CIRCULATION: 25ml sweet almond oil, 2 drops ylang-ylang, 2 drops petitgrain, 2 drops lemongrass, 4 drops coriander.

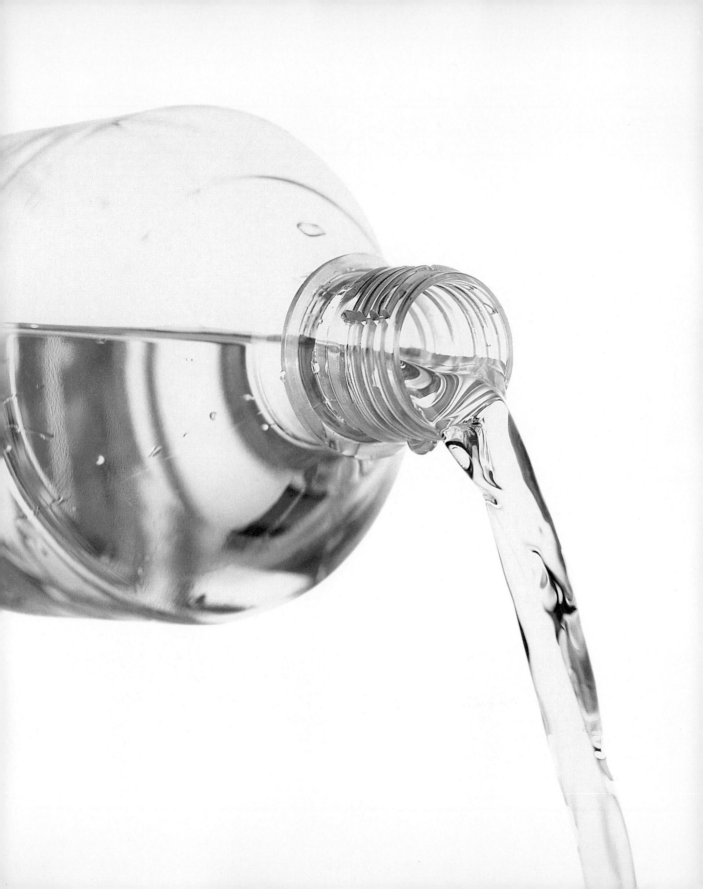

The Skin

The skin is the body's self-renewing outer covering and has many functions. Apart from the obvious job of keeping our insides together, it prevents excessive loss of water, salts and organic substances; regulates body temperature through perspiration; manufactures vitamin D from the sun and is the vehicle of our sense of touch and pain. It also expands and contracts, in a sense, 'breathes', excreting waste matter through the pores and acting as the body's first line of defence against chemical and bacterial agents. Indeed, the skin is an essential part of the immune system. It is laced with Langerhans cells which interact with the body's helper T cells (a type of white blood cell) to assist the body's immune responses. The skin is also capable of absorption, a function which is of special importance to aromatherapy.

Skin health is largely dependent upon its ability to maintain a reservoir of fluid; but up to two litres of moisture a day is lost through the pores, both as perspiration and, less noticably, evaporation. Provided the skin is functioning normally, evaporation of moisture is steadily replenished by its natural lipid secretions (a mix of oil and water) known as the skin's 'acid mantle'.

Even though conventional skin specialists recognize that anxiety and stress can trigger skin reactions (or exacerbate an existing skin problem), they persist in treating the skin locally as though it were a separate entity. For example, they may prescribe antibiotics to clear up acne or hydrocortisone cream to calm eczema. The danger with this approach is that, by suppressing the condition without addressing the possible causes, the ailment may go deeper and perhaps manifest later as a more serious complaint such as asthma, arthritis or weakened immunity.

It is essential, therefore, to be careful when attempting home treatment of skin complaints. If the underlying cause is not dealt with (be it a hidden food intolerance, chronic constipation or prolonged stress), aromatherapy can offer no more than temporary improvement. Long-term use of essential oils may even exacerbate the condition by triggering sensitization reactions.

For deep-rooted skin problems such as eczema, psoriasis and the kind of acne that has continued well into adulthood, it's essential to seek professional advice, perhaps from an accredited medical herbalist, homoeopathic practitioner or nutritionist.

Bearing this in mind, here are some effective treatments for a number of conditions affecting the skin and scalp. (For general skincare advice refer to the chart on pages 18 and 19.)

Good nutrition is essential for healthy skin

Acne

This common condition often begins at puberty when hormonal activity stimulates the sebaceous glands to secrete excess sebum, which causes spots, blackheads and boils. Some women notice that their acne gets worse prior to menstruation.

Although faulty nutrition is not the sole cause of acne, the complaint can certainly be made worse by a junk food diet washed down with excessive amounts of alcohol, tea and coffee. So cut back on these and drink plenty of bottled or filtered water, along with herb teas such as nettle, dandelion and horsetail which are rich in skin-healing nutrients. It can also be beneficial to take a daily multi-vitamin and mineral supplement containing 15mg of zinc and 800mg of vitamin A. Ideally, however, seek the advice of a holistic nutritionist who will devise a supplement programme tailored to your specific needs.

Carefully chosen essential oils can help control the condition if used as an adjunct to a healthy diet. Avoid the temptation to pick pustules as this may result in scarring. For daily cleansing, use a gentle soap-free cleansing bar (available from pharmacies and health shops). Soap can be too alkaline for some skins and may cause irritation. Since acne is associated with blockage of the follicles by sebum, have a steam facial and deep-cleansing face pack once or twice a week to open the pores (see the advice given for Spotty Skin, opposite). The following aromatic treatment will also be helpful.

◖ Aromatic Acne Lotion

The full-strength treatment is especially helpful if spots are oozing. Apply twice daily for 10 days, then, as the condition improves, reduce the quantity of essential oil by half and continue for a further 10 days. After this time, take a break from the oils and use a simple lotion such as distilled witch hazel or diluted cider vinegar (one part vinegar to eight parts water) for two to three weeks, before resuming with aromatherapy. Occasionally you may need to return to the full-strength blend for a few days to keep bacteria at bay. If you cannot obtain myrtle oil, tea tree may be substituted.

Full-Strength Lotion

10ml cider vinegar
2 drops frankincense essential oil
4 drops lavender essential oil
2 drops myrtle essential oil
125ml distilled water

Reduced-Strength Lotion

10ml cider vinegar
1 drop frankincense essential oil
2 drops lavender essential oil
1 drop myrtle essential oil
125ml distilled water

Funnel the cider vinegar into a dark glass bottle, then add the essential oils and shake well to disperse the oil. Top up with distilled water and shake again. Remember to shake each time before use. Apply with damp cotton wool pads.

 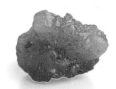

Frankincense can be very helpful in treating acne

Spotty Skin

Although not as widespread and persistent as full-blown acne, the problem can affect anyone beyond the age of puberty. An eruption of spots or pimples is more common in people with oily skin, especially during periods of emotional disharmony. Even the person with the finest complexion, however, is likely to experience the occasional outbreak of spots.

Try to eat at least five varied portions of fruit and vegetables daily; they contain antioxidants which promote clear skin and good health. Ideally these should be organic, and therefore pesticide-free, but if this is not possible then wash (and, where appropriate, peel) everything first. Drink a couple of mugfuls of warm bottled or filtered water each morning before or after breakfast to flush out your system and help prevent constipation.

It is important to cleanse your skin twice daily using a gentle soap-free cleansing bar. If you need to dry out a troublesome isolated spot, dab with undiluted calendula tincture or neat tea tree oil. Apply the tincture with a cotton bud, being careful to avoid the surrounding skin. To quell a cluster of spots, try one of the following aromatic treatments.

◗ Zit-Zapping Gel
For this healing potion, antiseptic and bactericidal essential oils are blended with anti-inflammatory aloe vera gel. Aloe vera is quickly absorbed without clogging the pores. For this reason, it can also be used as a daily moisturizer (without the addition of essential oils) for problem skin.

25ml aloe vera gel
1 drop tea tree
1 drop lavender

Put the aloe vera gel into a spotlessly clean cosmetic jar, then stir in the essential oils until thoroughly mixed. To ensure that the essential oils retain their maximum potency, don't be tempted to make larger quantities. The amount suggested here should be enough to last for seven to 10 days. After this time, make a fresh batch if necessary. Apply the gel two or three times a day after cleansing, for as long as required.

◗ Facial Sauna for Congested Skin
Most skins benefit from a deep-cleansing steam treatment once or twice a week, especially congested or oily skin that is prone to spots and blackheads.

Begin by cleansing your skin in the normal way. To prepare the facial sauna, fill a heatproof mixing bowl with near boiling water, then add two or three drops of any of the following essential oils: lavender, tea tree, frankincense, juniper berry, lemongrass, rosemary.

Hold your head over the steam and cover your head and the bowl with a towel to trap the aromatic vapours. Stay there for

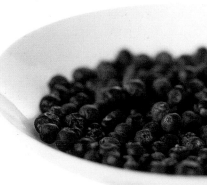

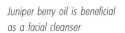

Juniper berry oil is beneficial as a facial cleanser

about five minutes. Afterwards, splash your face with tepid water to remove wastes accumulated on the skin's surface. You might like to follow this treatment with a face pack.

◗ Deep-Cleansing Clay Pack

This combination of green clay, yoghurt and frankincense has a deep cleansing, antiseptic and anti-inflammatory action on the skin, and is perfect for troublesome complexions. For best results, apply once or twice a week, immediately after a facial sauna while the skin is still warm and moist and, therefore, more receptive to whatever is applied to it.

3 level teaspoons fine green clay
3 teaspoons live, organic yoghurt (unflavoured)
1 drop frankincense essential oil

Mix the ingredients together to form a smooth paste. Smooth over your face and throat, avoiding the delicate eye area. Leave on for 10 to 15 minutes, then rinse off with tepid water. Allow the skin to settle for about one hour before applying a light moisturizer such as unperfumed aloe vera gel.

Beeswax granules are used as the basis for both rose petal and orange blossom creams

Dry Flaky Skin

Skin dryness is caused by a lack of water in the top layer of the skin, a condition that occurs more frequently as we grow older, or as a result of prolonged exposure to sun and wind. To improve the skin's smoothness and ability to lock in moisture, supplement your diet with evening primrose oil (2 x 500mg daily). Drink lots of bottled or filtered water. Water plumps up skin cells from within and helps ease dry skin problems.

External moisturizers are, of course, useful too. The skin creams described below are superb natural moisturizers for day and/or night-time use. They can be applied to the face, hands, feet or other areas of parched skin. Although much heavier than the super-light mousse creations available at the cosmetics counter, both products melt on contact with the skin. You will find a tiny amount will go a long way.

To prevent your skin from becoming too accustomed to one product, and therefore less responsive to its therapeutic effects, apply the rose cream once or twice daily for four to six weeks. After this time, switch to the orange blossom cream (or a shop-bought product) for the same length of time, before resuming with the rose cream. Continue cycling the treatment in this way for as long as required.

To enhance the skin's ability to retain moisture, apply the cream immediately after taking a bath or shower when it is still damp. Otherwise, put some spring water in a cosmetic bottle with a fine mist spray and spritz your skin.

◗ Rose Petal Skin Cream

7g beeswax granules (or grated beeswax
   if using a block)
25ml sweet almond oil
Contents of 3 x 500mg evening primrose
   oil capsules
30ml rosehip seed oil
30ml distilled water or rosewater
5 drops rose otto essential oil

*Put the beeswax and vegetable oils into a heatproof
bowl placed over a pan of simmering water. Warm
the distilled water in another bowl placed over another
pan of simmering water. Stir the beeswax and oil
mixture continuously until the beeswax has dissolved.
Remove the bowl from the heat and add the evening
primrose oil (pierce the capsules with a pin and
squeeze the contents into the mixture) and
stir well. Add the distilled water, a teaspoonful at a
time, while beating with a rotary whisk or electric mixer
set at the lowest speed. Keep beating until the cream
begins to thicken, then stir in the essential oil. Spoon
the mixture into little glass pots with tight-fitting lids.*

◗ Orange Blossom Skin Cream

7g beeswax granules (or grated beeswax if
   using a block)
15g cocoa butter
45ml sweet almond oil
35ml distilled water or orange flower water
5 drops neroli essential oil

*Put the beeswax, cocoa butter and sweet almond oil
into a heatproof bowl placed over a pan of simmering*

*water. Warm the distilled water in another bowl
placed over another pan of simmering water. Stir the
beeswax, cocoa butter and oil mixture continuously
until the beeswax has completely dissolved. Remove
the bowl from the heat and slowly add the warmed
distilled water, a teaspoonful at a time, while beating
with a rotary whisk or electric mixer set at the lowest
speed. Keep beating until the cream begins to cool
and thicken, then stir in the essential oil.*

◗ Honey and Avocado Face Pack

Honey is a marvellous moisturising agent, while
avocado contains a rich skin-softening oil. As an
alternative to mashed avocado in this recipe, you
may prefer to mix the honey with a couple of
teaspoons of avocado oil.

1 teaspoon liquid honey
2 teaspoons mashed avocado

*Mix together to form a smooth paste, then apply to
your face and neck. Leave on for 15 to 20 minutes,
before rinsing off with tepid water.*

STORAGE ADVICE

As these creams contain water, they are
vulnerable to developing mould. However, they
will usually keep for two or three months if
stored in a refridgerator or cool larder. To
ensure maximum shelf-life, avoid dipping
your fingers in the cream; use a teaspoon
or cosmetic spatula instead.

Chapped Lips

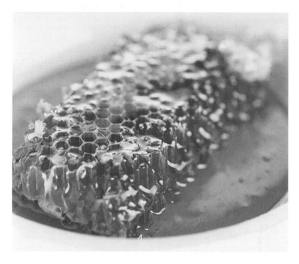

Honey is great for softening chapped lips

There are several different types of skin that cover the face and body. Our facial skin is the finest, but the thinnest skin of all is found on the lips, which is why they are so vulnerable to splitting and chapping in cold weather.

◉ Honey and Rose Lip Balm

This deliciously flavoured lip balm takes only a few minutes to make. It will moisturize, soften and protect your lips beautifully.

1 teaspoon beeswax granules (or 2 teaspoons grated beeswax if using a block)
3 teaspoons jojoba
1 teaspoon castor oil
½ teaspoon runny honey
1 drop rose otto essential oil

Put the beeswax, jojoba, castor oil and honey in a heatproof basin over a pan of simmering water.

Stir continuously until the beeswax has completely dissolved. Remove from the heat, add the essential oil and stir thoroughly. Pour the mixture into a little glass pot with a tight-fitting lid.

◉ Calendula and Chamomile Lip Salve

If your lips have become sore and cracked, try this healing salve.

1 teaspoon beeswax granules
 (or 2 teaspoons grated beeswax if using a block)
4 teaspoons macerated calendula oil
½ teaspoon runny honey
1 drop Roman chamomile essential oil

Put the beeswax, calendula oil and honey in a heat-proof basin over a pan of simmering water. Stir the mixture continuously until the beeswax has completely dissolved. Remove from the heat, add the essential oil and stir thoroughly. Pour the mixture into a little glass pot with a tight-fitting lid.

STORAGE ADVICE

As these products do not contain water, they have a shelf-life of three to four months. However, it's important to check regularly for signs of mould. They freeze well if stored in plastic containers and you may wish to save time by making a double quantity for long term use.

Boils

The cause of these inflamed pus-filled swellings on the skin is usually a bacterial infection in a hair follicle or a wound. They are usually painful to the touch and can be embarrassing, especially when they are on the face and neck. A tendency to develop boils indicates a run-down state in general, perhaps caused by poor nutrition or prolonged emotional stress. If you suffer from persistent boils have a medical check up, then perhaps consider holistic treatment from a medical herbalist, homoeopath or nutritionist.

To treat boils at home, the aromatherapy method consists of applications of hot and then cold compresses to draw out the boil. This is followed by an ointment or lotion to prevent the spread of infection.

● Hot and Cold Compresses (once or twice daily)

Start with a hot compress: Add four drops of German chamomile to 300ml of tolerably hot water. Soak a piece of folded gauze in the aromatic water then remove and apply to the boil. Hold in place until it cools, then reapply.

Finish with a cold compress: Add four drops of German chamomile to 300ml of cold water, then proceed as for a hot compress, holding in place until it warms to body temperature.

● Aromatic Ointment

This ointment is based on Hypercal which is available from pharmacies. Alternatively, make your own version (see Cold Sores, page 50).

25g Hypercal ointment
1 drop German chamomile essential oil
2 drops rosemary essential oil

Put the Hypercal ointment into a little pot, add the essential oils and stir well. Apply three times a day.

● Aromatic Lotion

If you prefer, use this lotion instead of the aromatic ointment described above.

25ml distilled witch hazel
25ml distilled water
1 drop German chamomile essential oil
2 drops lavender essential oil

Put the essential oils into a dark glass bottle, add the witch hazel and shake well. Top up with distilled water. Shake the bottle each time before use to disperse the oil. Apply with damp cotton wool pads. Repeat every few hours for as long as necessary.

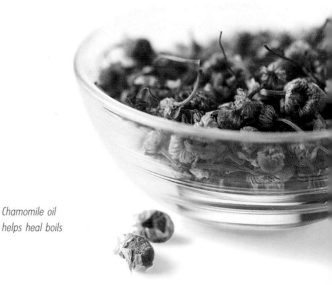

Chamomile oil helps heal boils

Stretch Marks

Although stretch marks occur frequently on the abdomen, breasts, buttocks and thighs of women who have been pregnant, they can also appear on the skin of anyone – male or female – who has suddenly gained weight. The marks first appear as reddish lines, gradually fading to white streaks resembling scar tissue. Once the marks have developed, it is impossible to eradicate them – although they can be prevented by combining applications of carefully selected oils.

Anti-Stretch Mark Blends

To prevent the possibility of a skin reaction from over-use of a particular essential oil (especially if used throughout pregnancy), use the following recipes in rotation. Apply the Calendula Smoothie blend for a month, the essential oil-free Butter-Up formula for the next month, then the Roses and Silk blend for a third month, resuming with the original formula, and so on.

Calendula Smoothie

30ml macerated calendula oil
20ml jojoba oil
6 drops mandarin
   essential oil
3 drops neroli essential oil
3 drops lavender essential oil

Put the calendula and jojoba oils into a dark glass bottle, add the essential oils and shake well.

Butter-Up

30g cocoa butter
20ml sweet almond oil

Melt the cocoa butter in a heatproof bowl placed over a pan of simmering water. Stir in the sweet almond oil. Remove from the heat and pour into a small jar. The mixture will harden slightly, but melts on contact with the skin.

Roses and Silk

25ml rosehip seed oil
25ml sweet almond oil
Contents of 2 vitamin E capsules
6 drops rose otto essential oil
 (or 5 drops geranium essential oil)
3 drops lavender essential oil

Put the rosehip seed and sweet almond oils into a dark glass bottle. Pierce the vitamin E capsules with a pin, then squeeze the contents into the mixture. Add the essential oils and shake well.

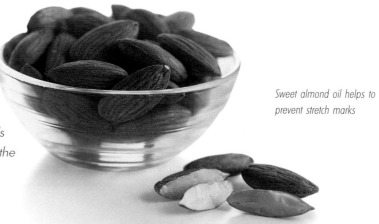

Sweet almond oil helps to prevent stretch marks

Nappy Rash

When a baby's skin is exposed to a wet or soiled nappy for too long it can become red, sore and irritated. Nappy rash can also be caused by acidic urine or stools; for example, after your baby has been given fruit (especially apples) or undiluted juice. Teething difficulties can also upset a baby's sensitive digestive system. An acidic internal state can be neutralized by giving your baby enough cooled, boiled water to drink.

Although oils such as chamomile and lavender are often recommended, they may further irritate a baby's delicate skin if used every day. Far better to apply a preventative proprietary zinc and castor oil cream. Should a rash develop, try applying the gentle ointment recommened below. Ensure your baby's skin is allowed to breathe by leaving off the nappy for at least one hour a day (with protective covering for the carpet or cot!).

Use a gentle cream to calm nappy rash

30g unperfumed skin cream
10ml macerated calendula oil
10ml macerated hypericum oil

Put the unperfumed skin cream into a cosmetic pot, add the macerated oils and stir until thoroughly mixed. Apply after every nappy change until the rash has cleared. Afterwards, continue with zinc and castor oil cream as a preventative.

Dandruff

Everyone's scalp flakes, but flaking is much increased when you have dandruff. It is the result of the scalp's skin cells drying out too fast as they move up from the reproductive layer to the skin's surface. In most cases, the presence of dandruff indicates insufficient rinsing after shampooing. Detergents and other chemicals found in most shampoos can irritate the scalp, thus resulting in increased flaking, if not completely rinsed out.

◊ Dandruff Treatment for Dry to Normal Hair

Wash your hair with a mild, pH-balanced shampoo, then towel dry. Massage your scalp with half of the mixture below, paying special attention to the ends which are prone to dryness and splitting. Cover your head with a towel and leave for up to an hour before shampooing again to remove the oil. To increase the effectiveness of the treatment, add cider vinegar to the final rinsing water (about three tablespoons to every two pints).

30ml extra virgin olive oil
2 drops rosemary essential oil
1 drop Roman chamomile essential oil
2 drops lavender essential oil
Contents of 2 x 500mg evening primrose
   oil capsules

This formula acts as an anti-dandruff and deep conditioning

Lavender for the treatment of dandruff

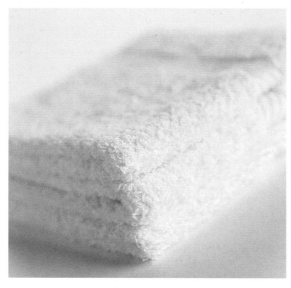

Towel dry your hair before applying dandruff treatments

15ml cider vinegar
3 drops Atlas cedarwood essential oil
3 drops rosemary essential oil
200ml distilled water

Funnel the cider vinegar into a dark glass bottle, then add the essential oils and shake well. Top up with distilled water and shake again. This should be sufficient for several applications.

⬥ Honey Hair and Scalp Pack

A conditioning and moisturizing treatment suitable for all hair types. It even helps clear stubborn cases of dandruff.

1½ tablespoons honey
3 teaspoons cider vinegar
3 drops lavender essential oil

Melt the honey in a heatproof bowl over a pan of simmering water. Remove from the heat and then stir in the cider vinegar and lavender oil. Massage the mixture into your scalp and then comb it through every part of your hair. Cover your head with a plastic shower cap and leave it on for up to one hour before shampooing out with a mild, pH-balanced shampoo.

treatment in one. A weekly application is usually enough to maintain a clear scalp and glossy hair. Unless your hair is very thick and long, the quantities given above should be enough for two treatments. Put the oils into a dark glass bottle. Pierce the evening primrose oil capsules with a pin and squeeze the contents into the mixture. Shake well.

⬥ Dandruff Treatment for Oily Hair

Wash your hair with a mild, pH-balanced shampoo, then towel dry. Pour a little hair tonic (below) into the palm of your hand and massage into the scalp and through the hair. There is no need to rinse.

You may find that if you use this product three times a week, the over-secretion of sebum will be reduced. The cider vinegar helps restore the skin's natural acid mantle.

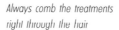

Always comb the treatments right through the hair

Headlice

Headlice live on the scalp and feed by sucking blood. Their bites cause itching and scratching which can lead to scalp infections and dermatitis. The lice are spread by head-to-head contact, especially between young children at school. Headlice eggs (nits) glue to the hair shafts and are difficult to see. If overused, organophosphorous compounds in conventional headlice preparations may be toxic to the nervous system and are potentially carcinogenic. Although containing quite a high concentration of essential oils, the following tried and tested treatment not only smells good, but is safe and effective for all school-age children. It also improves the quality of the hair rather than damaging it.

PREVENTATIVE MEASURES AGAINST HEADLICE

During an outbreak, add five drops of lavender or tea tree oil to 20ml of an unperfumed shampoo and use this regularly, as headlice are repelled by the aroma. Remember, if a child has headlice, it is a good idea to treat the whole family in case of cross-infection.

◖ Headlice Banishing Oil

100ml vegetable oil (for example, sunflower or olive)
10 drops eucalyptus
20 drops rosemary essential oil
20 drops lavender essential oil
10 drops geranium essential oil

Funnel the vegetable oil into a dark glass bottle, add the essential oils and shake well. Apply to wet hair (otherwise it will be difficult to shampoo out the oil) by massaging well into the scalp to reach the hair roots. Leave it on for at least one hour (preferably up to three hours) then shampoo thoroughly. Remove dead lice and nits with a regulation fine-toothed comb (essential oils destroy the lice but not the eggs). Repeat the treatment twice more at three-day intervals to ensure the infestation is completely cleared.

Geranium oil helps remove headlice

HOW TO USE A NIT COMB

You may be able to obtain one of the new battery-operated nit combs which kill the lice on contact. However, the traditional type does still remove nits. After carrying out the aromatic treatment given above, begin combing at the hairline at the back of the neck. Part the hair into very thin strands and comb through the entire lengths systematically, allowing at least 10 minutes for the task. Many nits stick close to the scalp, so pay special attention to the hair roots. After withdrawing the comb each time, wipe it with a tissue to remove the nits and dead lice, then discard the tissue immediately. When you have finished combing, it is a good idea to burn the used tissues.

Athlete's Foot

This highly infectious fungal infection thrives in warm, moist conditions like those in swimming pools and gym changing rooms. It affects the skin between and underneath the toes, causing it to become white, spongy, itchy and cracked. Whenever possible, expose afflicted feet to sunshine and fresh air. Wear leather shoes (open sandals in summer) and cotton socks which allow the skin to breathe.

The following aromatic prescriptions contain essential oils with fungicidal properties; all have been found effective for athlete's foot. One other plant-based remedy with fungicidal properties is calendula cream (available from health stores and pharmacies). This can be used by itself or boosted with the addition of appropriate essential oils.

◉ Aromatic Vinegar for Athlete's Foot

20ml cider vinegar
30ml distilled water or
   boiled water
3 drops lemongrass
   essential oil
3 drops tea tree essential oil
5 drops lavender
   essential oil

Funnel the cider vinegar into a dark glass bottle. Add the essential oils and shake well. Add the water and shake

again. You will need to shake well each time before use to disperse the oils. Using cotton wool, or cotton bud if only a tiny area is affected, and apply three times a day.

◉ Athlete's Foot Ointment

25g calendula cream
3 drops myrrh essential oil
3 drops lavender essential oil
1 drop patchouli essential oil

Put the calendula cream into a glass cosmetic pot, then add the essential oils. Using the handle of a teaspoon, stir until thoroughly mixed. Apply two or three times a day.

◉ Athlete's Foot Powder

3 tablespoons sifted rice flour (or cornflour)
10 drops lavender essential oil
3 drops lemongrass essential oil
10 drops tea tree essential oil

Put the rice flour into a glass jar, add the oils and shake. Cover the jar with a tight-fitting lid and allow the base to absorb the oils for 24 hours before applying. Use daily to powder the affected areas. It is also helpful to sprinkle the powder inside shoes to help prevent reinfection and to deodorize the footwear.

Calendula eases many skin conditions

Ringworm

Ringworm is a contagious fungal infection of the skin, which can be caught from pets. It appears as an inflamed itchy rash in circular patches anywhere on the body, including the scalp. This ring-like appearance gives the condition its name, so it has nothing to do with worms! If ringworm affects the scalp, hair loss can occur.

Scrupulous hygiene is essential to prevent the infection spreading. Do not share hairbrushes, combs, sheets, pillowcases or towels with an infected person. To boost your overall immunity to infection, add garlic, onions and fresh herbs such as thyme and rosemary to your food. A good quality multivitamin and mineral supplement may also be beneficial.

Garlic added to the diet boosts the immune system

For direct treatment, try one of the following aromatic preparations. These should be effective within 10 days; if not, seek professional help.

◗ Ringworm Ointment

30g unperfumed skin cream
 (available from pharmacies)
5ml calendula tincture
4 drops myrrh essential oil
8 drops lavender essential oil
4 drops lemongrass essential oil

Put the unperfumed skin cream into a little glass pot, then stir in the tincture and essential oils until thoroughly mixed. Apply three or four times daily.

◗ Aromatic Ringworm Lotion (for the scalp)

1 tablespoon cider vinegar
200ml distilled (or cool boiled) water
5 drops tea tree essential oil
2 drops peppermint essential oil
5 drops lavender essential oil

Put the cider vinegar into a dark glass bottle, add the essential oils and shake well. Top up with distilled water and shake again. Gently massage this mixture into the scalp twice a day, including after shampooing.

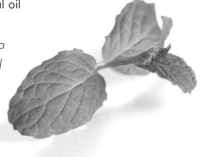

Peppermint essential oil helps alleviate ringworm

◗ Calendula and Myrrh Lotion (for skin and scalp)

If you have ringworm on both body and scalp, it may be easier to use this dual purpose lotion. Calendula and myrrh tinctures are available from herbal suppliers.

25ml calendula tincture
25ml myrrh tincture

Funnel the tinctures into a dark glass bottle and shake well. For treating ringworm on the body, apply undiluted three times a day (using damp cotton wool). For scalp treatment, add three teaspoons of the tincture to 30ml water and gently massage into the scalp twice a day, including after shampooing.

Cold Sores (Herpes Simplex)

Herpes of the mouth – or cold sores – are caused by the herpes simplex virus. The virus lies dormant in many people, flaring up during periods of stress or when the body becomes weakened through infections such as colds and flu. Sunlight on the skin can be a trigger in some people. The blister-like sores announce their arrival by tingling and itching and can last a week or more. According to many nutritionists, food intolerances are often implicated, especially foods containing the amino acid arginine which is found in chocolate, nuts, mushrooms, tomatoes, green peppers, pork, sunflower oil and shellfish such as crabs and shrimp. On the positive side, foods such as beansprouts, soya products, fish (especially halibut), poultry such as chicken and turkey (preferably free-range), yoghurt and brewer's yeast are rich in the amino acid lysine which is thought to suppress the herpes simplex virus.

At the first sign of cold sores, apply either of the ointments that are listed below. They can often quell an eruption within 24 hours.

Chocolate could be a trigger for cold sores

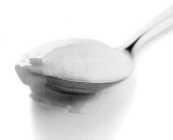

Yoghurt in the diet can help suppress cold sores

◖ Aromatic Hypercal Ointment

20g hypercal ointment (available from pharmacies)
2 drops German chamomile

Put the hypercal ointment into a small cosmetic pot, then stir in the essential oil using the handle of a teaspoon. Apply a little of the ointment to the affected area every few hours and continue to apply for as long as necessary.

◖ High-Strength Hypercal Ointment

Here is a simple recipe for making your own high-strength hypercal ointment. For many people this treatment is effective, even without the addition of essential oils.

25g unperfumed skin cream
  (available from pharmacies)
5ml hypericum tincture
5ml calendula tincture

Put the unperfumed skin cream into a little glass pot, then stir in the tinctures. Apply a little of the ointment to the affected area several times a day for as long as required.

Eczema

There are two main types of eczema: atopic (chronic or long-term) and contact dermatitis. The first is usually hereditary, associated with a family history of asthma, hay fever or migraine. Food intolerances may also be implicated, especially to dairy products. In contact dermatitis there may be a local reaction to household and industrial chemicals, certain plants (such as primrose), nickel, cosmetics, perfumes and even essential oils. Contact allergy is also highly likely to occur in people with atopic eczema.

Symptoms of both kinds of eczema include an itchy, red, painful (sometimes weepy) rash. In chronic cases, the skin may crack and bleed. For the reasons given at the start of this chapter, anyone who has eczema is advised, first of all, to seek professional help from a qualified homoeopath, medical herbalist or holistic nutritionist, ideally with the consent of a doctor.

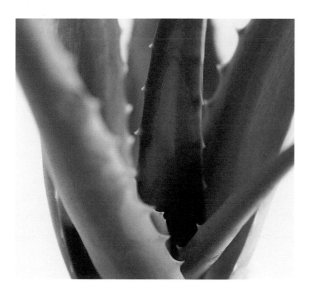

Aloe vera gel brings relief to eczema sufferers

As a general self-help measure, studies have shown that evening primrose oil is highly beneficial when taken as a nutritional supplement (6 x 500mg capsules daily). For some eczema sufferers, it can also be helpful to apply the oil externally. For many others, however, oil-based applications cause the skin to overheat, thus exacerbating the condition. The oil-free treatments suggested below will not cure eczema, but they will certainly reduce inflammation and itching.

◦ Calendula and Aloe Vera Gel (for dry eczema)

50ml aloe vera gel
15 drops calendula tincture

Put the aloe vera gel into a little glass pot, add the calendula tincture and stir well. Apply to the affected areas two or three times daily.

◦ Calendula Compress (for weepy eczema)

250ml bottled or filtered water
  (or cooled boiled tap water)
20 drops calendula tincture

Put the water into a bowl, add the calendula tincture and swish around to disperse. Soak a piece of clean, folded, cotton fabric in the water, wring out and apply to the affected area for 15 minutes.

Skin First Aid

SUNBURN

If the skin is very sore, making the application of ointments and gels painful, one of the most effective treatments for sunburn is to spray the skin with aloe vera juice. This is different from the cosmetic aloe vera gel used in previous recipes. Aloe vera juice is a nutritional supplement available from health stores. It will prevent sunburnt skin from peeling. It also takes out the heat and sting, stops blistering and converts minor sunburn into a tan. Put some into a cosmetic spray bottle and mist your skin several times a day. Otherwise, try one of the following aromatic treatments.

🜂 Cooling Bath

To soothe mild sunburn on large areas of the body, try this healing bath formula.

250ml cider vinegar
3 drops Roman (or German) chamomile
    essential oil
3 drops lavender essential oil

Mix the essential oils with the vinegar, then add to a cool, preferably cold, bath and swish around to disperse. Soak for about 15 minutes. Afterwards apply the cooling gel (below).

🜂 Cooling Gel

This healing gel combines the anti-inflammatory properties of aloe vera with the skin-regenerating properties of the essential oils. For the more sensitive

skin of the face, use half the quantity of essential oil in the recipe. You may need to make separate products for the face and body.

50ml aloe vera gel
2 drops rosemary
    essential oil
2 drops lavender
    essential oil
2 drops tea tree
    essential oil

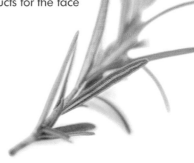
Rosemary helps heal sunburn

IMPORTANT: Extensive sunburn requires urgent medical attention.

BRUISES

When an injury damages tiny blood vessels under the skin, the surface appears discoloured and bruised. Occasional bumps and bruises can be treated easily at home, but frequent or widespread bruising, resulting from minor injury or no obvious cause, needs to be checked by a doctor. If you are prone to frequent bruising, it can be beneficial to supplement your diet with vitamin C (2 x 500mg daily) which is thought to strengthen the blood capillaries. To reduce swelling and speed up healing, try one of the following first-aid treatments.

🜂 Cold Compress to Reduce Bruising

600ml ice-cold water
3 drops sweet marjoram essential oil
3 drops Roman chamomile essential oil

Put the water into a bowl, then add the essential oils and swish around to disperse the oil. Soak a piece of clean, folded cotton fabric in the aromatic water, wring out and place over the bruised area. Leave in place until the fabric warms to body temperature. Reapply several times more, until pain is reduced.

Bruise Ointment

For best results, use this ointment after treatment with cold compresses (as above).

25g unperfumed skin cream
  (available from pharmacies)
5ml calendula tincture
2 drops helichrysum essential oil
2 drops Roman chamomile essential oil
3 drops lavender essential oil

Put the unperfumed skin cream into a little glass pot, then add the tincture and essential oils and stir until thoroughly mixed. Apply two or three times daily.

Healing Eye Gel (for a black eye)

For bruising around the eye, never apply essential oils; should any seep into the eyes, it may cause further pain and irritation. Instead, use an eye pad soaked in ice cold witch hazel for about 15 minutes, and then apply this healing gel.

20ml aloe vera gel
10 drops of calendula tincture

Put the aloe vera gel into a sterilized glass pot, add the calendula tincture and stir until thoroughly mixed.

Apply three times a day. Pat a little of the gel around the eye area, but away from the eye itself.

BURNS AND SCALDS (minor)

Before applying oils or ointments, it's essential to cool the burn under cold running water for 10 minutes or until the pain has gone. To cool larger areas of skin, stand under a tepid shower or get into a cool bath. After cooling the skin, apply neat lavender or tea tree oil if the burn is very small. For larger burns and scalds, apply one of the following aromatic formulas.

IMPORTANT: Do not puncture blisters as this may cause infection. If a burn becomes increasingly painful or infected, seek medical help.

Healing Oil for Burns and Scalds

20ml macerated calendula oil
20ml macerated hypericum oil
3 drops lavender (or tea tree) essential oil

Funnel the macerated oils into a dark glass bottle, add the essential oil and shake well to disperse. Smooth into the affected areas two or three times daily for as long as required.

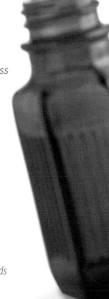

Use dark glass bottles for oil blends

◊ Ointment for Burns and Scalds

25g unperfumed skin cream
  (available from pharmacies)
5 drops frankincense essential oil
5 drops rosemary essential oil
5 drops lavender (or tea tree) essential oil

◊ Cold Compress for Burns and Scalds

300ml cold water
4 drops German chamomile (or tea tree, or lavender) essential oil

Put the water into a bowl, add the essential oil and swish around to disperse. Soak a gauze dressing in the aromatic water, wring out the excess and apply to the burn. Bandage the compress in place, then renew after a few hours. Repeat as often as necessary until pain and inflammation have subsided.

INSECT BITES AND STINGS

Some people are more vulnerable to bites and stings than others, probably because they smell delicious! Insects do not like the smell of garlic, so eating it can help keep them at bay. Mosquitoes and some other bugs are repelled by the taste of vitamin B. Try taking a 50mg vitamin B complex tablet every day for at least a week before going away. Should you still get attacked, here are some aromatic remedies to take the sting out of the holiday season.

◊ First-Aid Essentials for Insect Bites and Stings

Cider vinegar or fresh lemon juice
Lavender or tea tree essential oil
Bicarbonate of soda
Water
Tweezers

You can dab most bites and stings with a little neat lavender or tea tree oil, but wasp stings, which are alkaline, must first be neutralized with a dab of cider vinegar or lemon juice. Apply as often as necessary until the pain and swelling subside. A single drop of lavender or tea tree oil added to two teaspoons of cider vinegar or lemon juice helps prevent infection.

With bee stings first remove the stinger (a black hair-like structure left behind by the bee) with a pair of tweezers. Hold the tweezers as near to the skin as possible to avoid squeezing the venom sac, which will pump more poison into the body. Bee and ant venom, which are acidic, can be neutralized with bicarbonate of soda. Mix one rounded teaspoon into a paste with a little water and add a drop of lavender or tea tree oil to prevent infection.

IMPORTANT: Bee and wasp stings affect some people seriously. If the person stung feels faint, or has difficulty breathing, summon urgent medical attention.

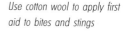

Use cotton wool to apply first aid to bites and stings

CUTS AND GRAZES

Carefully swab the wound with wet cotton wool or hold the injured part under running water until the bleeding stops. Deep wounds may need stitching, so if you are unsure it might be best to consult a doctor.

IMPORTANT: If the cut has been caused by a rusty nail, barbed wire or animal bite, or has been in contact with the soil, you may need a tetanus shot, so contact your doctor. While awaiting medical attention, swab the affected area with a strong solution of hypericum tincture: four teaspoons of tincture to a teacupful of water. Although it may not be advisable to trust the remedy entirely, in ancient times hypericum was used to prevent tetanus in soldiers wounded in battle.

For less serious injuries, having cleansed the wound, natural remedies will encourage healing and help to prevent scarring. Simply apply neat lavender or tea tree oil, or try one of the following aromatic treatments.

⬩ Cold Aromatic Compress

600ml water
2 drops eucalyptus (or tea tree) essential oil
2 drops lemon essential oil
2 drops lavender essential oil

Put the water in a bowl, add the essential oils and swish around to disperse. Soak a clean piece of folded cotton fabric in the water, wring out the excess and apply to the wound. Hold the compress in place for 10 minutes. *Afterwards, if necessary, cover the wound with a bandage or plaster to protect it.*

⬩ Antiseptic Ointment

For this recipe, instead of using unperfumed skin cream as a base, you may prefer to add the essential oils to a proprietary hypercal ointment. If so you will need to omit the calendula and hypericum tinctures.

25g unperfumed skin cream
  (available from pharmacies)
5ml calendula tincture
5ml hypericum tincture
3 drops frankincense essential oil
2 drops myrrh essential oil
4 drops lavender essential oil

Put the unperfumed skin cream into a little glass pot. Add the tinctures and essential oils and stir until thoroughly mixed. Apply the ointment two or three times a day for as long as necessary.

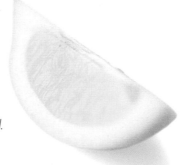

Lemon essential oil encourages healing

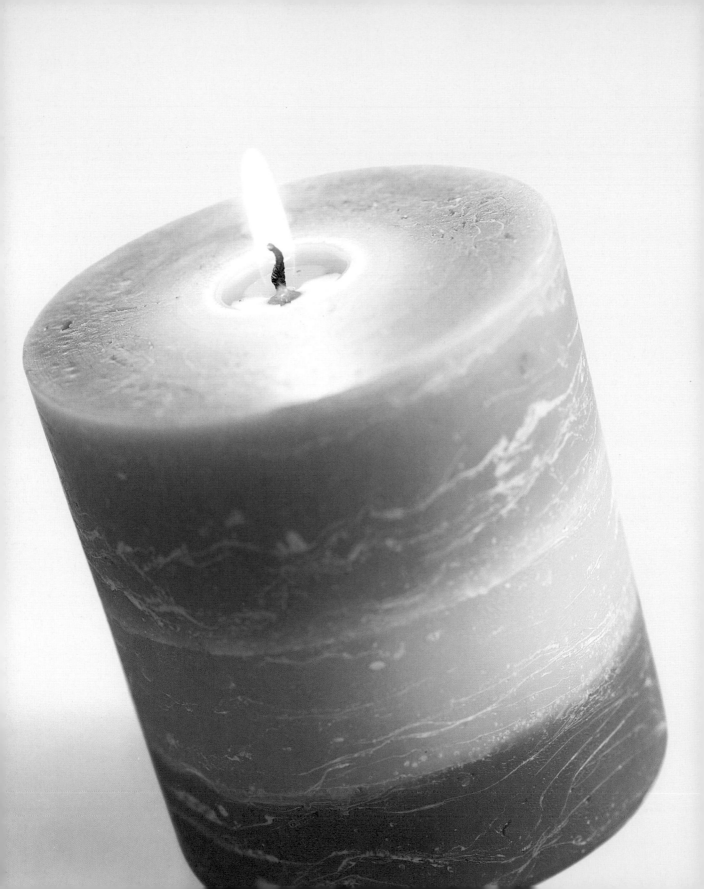

The Respiratory System

Supplying the cells with life-giving oxygen is the shared responsibility of the respiratory and circulatory systems. And since the lungs share the role of eliminating waste with the skin, kidneys and colon, if a problem develops in any of these systems the body compensates by increasing the burden on the others.

It is important to clarify the terms breathing and respiration. Breathing is the movement of air in and out of the lungs by means of the diaphragm (situated beneath the rib cage) and intercostal muscles (situated between the ribs). Respiration is the chemical process occuring inside all living cells whereby nutrients are oxidized to produce energy, and carbon dioxide and other tissue wastes are eliminated from the system.

Respiratory ailments affect the mucous membranes. These include the linings of the nose, sinuses, mouth, throat, windpipe and lungs. The fine coverings of the eyes and the linings of certain parts of the inner ear are also covered by mucus-producing membranes. When health is compromised, perhaps through poor diet, emotional disharmony or cigarette smoke, we become more susceptible to bacterial and viral infection.

The aim of natural treatment is not only to alleviate symptoms with gentle remedies, but also to strengthen the immune defences through improved nutrition, adequate exercise, breathing exercises and relaxation techniques. The last three elements can be embraced through yoga, you may wish to find out about classes in your area.

Certain dietary measures can be taken to help build your resistence to common respiratory ailments such as coughs, colds and flu. Cut down on sugar, chemical-laden junk food, dairy products, and foods made from white flour, as these encourage the body to produce excess mucus (catarrh). Increase your intake of fresh fruit and vegetables – preferably organic and therefore free of pesticide residues – including garlic, onions and leeks, to help combat chest infections. It can also help to take garlic supplements (available from health stores) and to use herbs and spices such as rosemary, cinnamon, thyme and ginger in your cooking, as these help to clear your chest.

Enhance your immune system with herbs such as thyme

IMPORTANT: The management and treatment of serious respiratory conditions such as asthma, chronic bronchitis and emphysema require medical intervention. If you are concerned about the condition of a baby, young child or elderly person, please seek medical advice.

Bronchitis

Bronchitis is inflammation of the mucous lining of the bronchial tree (the tubes to the lungs). It can be acute (short-term) or chronic (long-term). It is defined as a persistent phlegm-producing cough lasting more than three months. Acute bronchitis can result from infection after a cold or flu. Symptoms are a chesty cough, wheezing, high temperature and chest pain.

As well as the treatments suggested in this section, herb teas such as elderflower, yarrow and elecampane are excellent remedies. If the condition tends to come on during cold, damp weather – and if the sputum is white and copious, try the spicy drink recommended for colds (opposite).

◗ Essential Oil Concentrate for Bronchitis Treatments

Here is a concentrated mixture of decongestant essential oils. The blend is measured by the drop for use in steam inhalations and baths, and for making a chest rub. A few drops of the concentrate may also be put on to a tissue and inhaled at intervals throughout the day.

15 drops Atlas cedarwood essential oil
15 drops frankincense essential oil
12 drops Canadian balsam (or Scots pine)
  essential oil
8 drops myrrh essential oil

Put the essential oils into a small dark glass bottle, then shake well. Dispense the mixture (as directed below) using a pipette (eye dropper) which can be obtained from your local pharmacy.

Steam Inhalation: *Add four drops of the concentrate to a bowl of almost boiling water, two drops for children over five years. Cover your head and the bowl with a towel to form a tent and inhale the aromatic vapour for five minutes. Carry out the treatment two to three times daily.*

CAUTION: Avoid steam inhalations if you have asthma; concentrated steam may trigger an attack. Instead, you may derive benefit from aromatic baths.

Aromatic Bath: *A supportive treatment to be used as an adjunct to the more powerfully decongestant steam inhalation. Whenever you take a bath, add eight drops of the concentrate to the water, four drops for children over five years.*

Chest and Back Rub: *Use in combination with the steam inhalation. For adults, add 15 drops of concentrate to 25ml vegetable base oil (such as sunflower, sweet almond or olive). For children over five years, use seven drops of concentrate to 25ml base oil. Apply twice a day.*

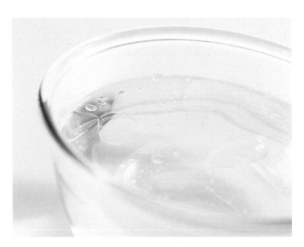

Steam inhalations can help bronchitis

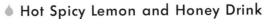

Colds

A cold is an upper respiratory viral infection affecting the nasal passages and throat. There are many different cold viruses around and new strains are evolving constantly. So even though you develop immunity to a particular cold virus once you catch it, there is always another version ready to reinfect you. Stress of any kind can weaken the immune system, leaving you vulnerable to passing cold (and flu) viruses. As a preventative measure, most natural health experts recommend vitamin C supplements (2 x 500mg daily) which help strengthen the immune defences. Should you still catch a cold, the following aromatic treatments can help reduce symptoms and shorten a cold's duration.

◆ Essential Oil Concentrate for Treating Colds

15 drops eucalyptus essential oil
  (or use myrtle oil for children under 10 years)
15 drops sweet marjoram essential oil
10 drops lavender essential oil
10 drops rosemary essential oil

Put the essential oils into a small dark glass bottle and shake well. Use as recommended for bronchitis (opposite).

◆ Hot Spicy Lemon and Honey Drink

If taken at the first sign of cold or flu symptoms (such as sore throat, shivering and sneezing), this spicy brew may even stop the virus from developing further. It is also helpful for acute bronchitis (opposite).

600ml water
1 teaspoon whole cloves
¼ cinnamon stick, broken
1 teaspoon grated dried ginger root
  (or 2 teaspoons if using fresh ginger root)
Honey according to taste
Juice of one freshly squeezed lemon
Scant sprinkling of ground cayenne pepper
  (optional)

Pour the water into a stainless steel or enamel saucepan, add the spices (except the cayenne pepper) and simmer in a covered pan for 20 minutes. To make a teacupful of the spicy drink, put three teaspoons of lemon juice into the cup, then top up with the spicy brew. Sweeten with honey according to taste. Add a touch of cayenne pepper if you dare (very fiery!). Take one teacupful three times a day.

The mixture can be gently re-heated to just below simmering point each time before use. If the spices are left seeping in the pan of water, the mixture will continue to increase in strength. So add a teacupful of water to the pan each time it is re-heated. However, make a fresh batch after 24 hours – that is, if you still need the remedy!

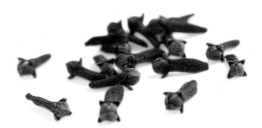

Add whole cloves to the Hot Spicy Lemon and Honey Drink to ward off colds and flu

Influenza (flu)

Influenza is a viral infection affecting the nasal passages and throat, causing fever, headache, general aches and pains, nasal congestion, fatigue and depression. Symptoms tend to ease within four to five days, though general weakness may persist for a few weeks. There are many different flu viruses, including new strains which appear every decade or so. Elderly people, babies and young children are at greatest risk of becoming seriously ill with flu. In such cases, medical advice is essential.

Loss of appetite is common during a bout of flu, so do not force yourself to eat. Instead, drink plenty of bottled water, fruit juices diluted 50:50 with water, and herb teas such as peppermint, thyme and elderflower (see also the advice given for colds, page 59). Essential oil treatments will ease symptoms, lift your spirits and prevent any serious complications.

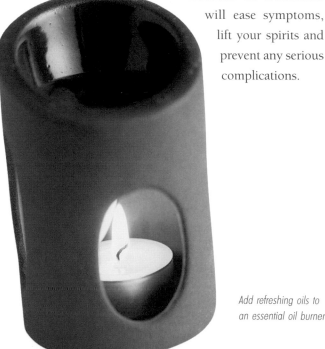

Add refreshing oils to an essential oil burner

● Essential Oil Concentrate for Flu Symptoms

10 drops rosemary essential oil
10 drops coriander essential oil
10 drops sweet marjoram essential oil
10 drops mandarin essential oil
10 drops eucalyptus essential oil
  (or use myrtle for children under 10)

Put the essential oils into a dark glass bottle and shake well. Use as recommended for bronchitis (page 58).

● Aromatic Fumigant

To purify the air during flu epidemics, vaporize this high-strength mixture of refreshing oils.

3 drops Canadian balsam (or Scots pine) essential oil
3 drops Atlas cedarwood essential oil
3 drops juniper berry essential oil
5 drops lemon essential oil

Add the essential oils to the water-filled reservoir, then light the candle. If using an electric vaporizer or diffuser, make sure you follow the manufacturer's instructions. If you do not have a purpose-designed gadget, add the essential oils to a plant mister containing about 200ml of water. Spray every room in your home at least twice a day.

Coughs

A cough is the body's attempt to clear air passages of external irritants or symptoms of a cold, flu, bronchitis or a more serious condition like asthma.

As part of the treatment avoid dairy products and refined starches. The Hot Spicy Lemon and Honey Drink recommended for colds (see page 59) is a wonderful remedy for coughs as well.

IMPORTANT: A persistent cough must be investigated by a doctor, perhaps followed by holistic treatment from a medical herbalist or homoeopath.

● Essential Oil Concentrate for Coughs

10 drops cypress essential oil
15 drops lavender essential oil
10 drops frankincense essential oil
10 drops myrtle (or rosemary) essential oil

Put the essential oils into a dark glass bottle and shake well. Use as recommended for bronchitis (see page 58).

● Gargle for Coughs

2 teaspoons cider vinegar
2 drops sweet marjoram essential oil
1 teacup warm water
½ teaspoon runny honey

Put the cider vinegar into a teacup. Add the essential oils, then top up with warm water and stir in the honey. Use two or three times a day.

Sinusitis

This is an infection of the sinus cavities resulting in nasal congestion, pain around the eyes, headaches and sometimes bad breath as well. If not treated properly, the condition can develop into a chronic complaint causing almost constant discomfort. If you are prone to sinusitis, it is advisable to seek constitutional treatment from a medical herbalist or homoeopath. For an occasional attack of sinusitis, you will find the following treatment helpful.

● Essential Oil Concentrate for Sinusitis Treatment

This concentrated mixture of decongestant and pain-relieving essential oils is most effective when used in steam inhalations – as recommended for the treatment of bronchitis (see page 58). In addition, a few drops may be put onto a tissue and inhaled as required throughout the day.

10 drops peppermint essential oil
15 drops lavender essential oil
10 drops eucalyptus essential oil

Put the essential oils into a dark glass bottle and shake well.

CAUTION: Peppermint and eucalyptus oils may cause breathing problems in children under seven years of age.

Hayfever

This is a seasonal allergy to airborne pollens. It is characterized by sneezing, a blocked or runny nose, itchy, streaming eyes, sensitivity to light and a 'heavy' head. Some people also develop a fever or suffer asthma-like symptoms such as coughing and wheezing.

In an allergic person, the body's defence system reacts to pollen as if it were poison, so it produces antibodies which interact with pollen leading to the release of histamine and other chemicals. From this, it may be easier to understand why natural treatment for hayfever is a complex all-body concern, involving dietary reform and de-stressing techniques. The home treatments suggested here will certainly ease symptoms, but for complete relief it is advisable to consult a medical herbalist, homoeopath or holistic nutritionist. Such a practitioner will be able to devise a treatment plan tailored to your specific needs.

It can be helpful to take two teaspoons of local honey from the honeycomb daily for six weeks before your symptoms usually begin. The pollen grains in it can help desensitize you to pollens in your area. Nutritionists advise taking a vitamin C supplement with added bioflavonoids (500mg three times daily), which acts as a natural antihistimine. Elderflower and eyebright herbal teas will help clear catarrh (take as directed on the label). You can also use cooled eyebright tea to bathe sore, itchy eyes. A number of essential oils are potentially helpful for hayfever. However, because individual reactions vary according to the oil, you will need to experiment until you find the oil(s) most compatible with your own body. Try one oil at a time, chosen from the following: rose otto (the most expensive!), eucalyptus, chamomile (German or Roman), Canadian balsam, frankincense, lavender, peppermint or tea tree. Apply using the same methods and overall quantities as for bronchitis (page 58). You may also find the following remedy helpful.

● Hayfever Balm

Although not a 'natural' substance, the petroleum jelly in this recipe merely acts as a carrier for the essential oil. It can evaporate and enter the nasal cavities without being absorbed into the skin. It will also trap dust and pollen which trigger attacks.

1 teaspoon petroleum jelly
1–2 drops essential oil
  (use whichever oil works best for you)

Put the petroleum jelly into a little glass pot, then stir in the essential oil. Apply a very small amount to the nostrils two or three times daily.

CAUTION: Avoid peppermint and eucalyptus oils on children under seven years, as these may cause breathing difficulties.

Eucalyptus oil can help alleviate hayfever

Throat Problems

A sore throat is often the first symptom of a cold or flu virus, or some other viral infection. Laryngitis is inflammation of the larynx (voice box) resulting in huskiness and weakness of the voice and sometimes a dry cough. It often results from overuse of the voice and is common in public speakers, singers and actors. Whatever the cause of a throat problem, try the following treatment.

◆ Aromatic Gargle

1 teacupful warm water
1 teaspoon cider vinegar
1 drop lemon essential oil
1 drop eucalyptus essential oil
½ teaspoon honey

Put the cider vinegar into a teacup, then stir in the essential oils. Top up with warm water and stir in the honey. Use two or three times daily.

IMPORTANT: Recurrent or persistent sore throats which do not appear to be associated with inflammation or infection may be an early sign of a thyroid disorder. So a medical check-up is strongly advised.

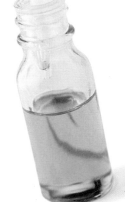

Add ear drops morning and night

Earache

Earache can occur as a secondary infection in children who have a viral or bacterial infection in the nose or throat. Recurrent ear infections need to be investigated by a doctor, medical herbalist or homoeopath. The following aromatic treatments will help ease pain and resolve the infection.

CAUTION: Pus or a bloody discharge indicates something more serious. Seek urgent medical attention.

◆ Aromatic Ear Drops

1–2 drops German chamomile
  (or rosemary) essential oil
1 teaspoon sweet almond oil

Put the sweet almond oil into an egg cup, then stir in the essential oil. Using a pipette, put a few drops into the ear and plug with cotton wool. Do this in the morning and at bedtime for as long as necessary.

◆ Aromatic Compress for Earache

This method can be used in conjunction with the previous method, though it is often effective by itself.

600ml (1pt) comfortably hot water
4 drops German chamomile (or rosemary) essential oil

Pour the water into a bowl, add the essential oil and swish around to disperse. Soak a piece of cotton fabric in the water, then ring out the excess. Hold the compress in place until it has cooled to body temperature. Replenish the compress two or three times in succession.

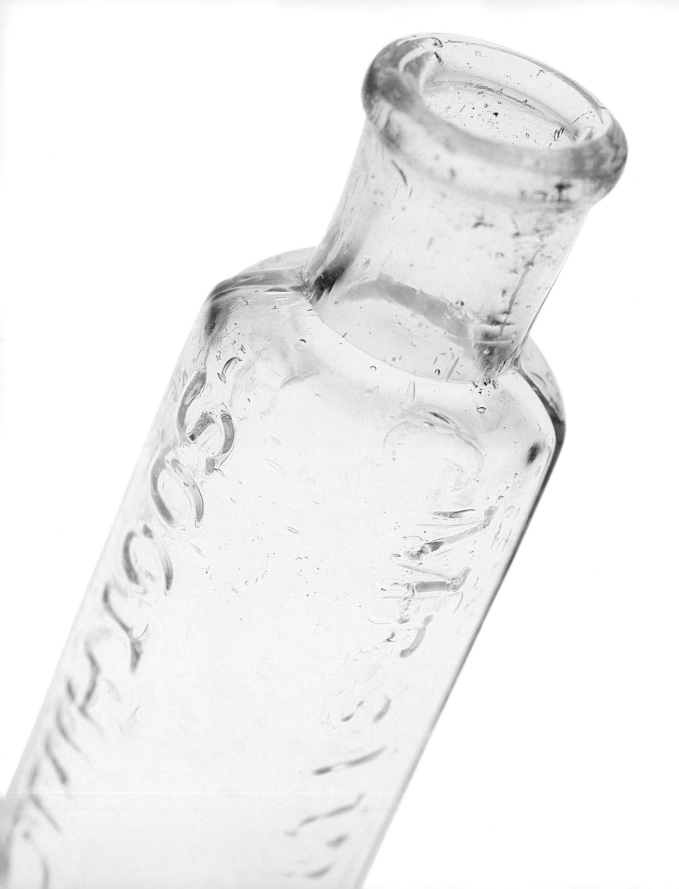

The Heart and Circulation

Every cell in the body needs a constant supply of blood to bring in oxygen and nutrients. If the supply is insufficient, we experience a marked decrease in vitality.

The average adult has six litres (10 pints) of blood circulating in the body. The force (blood pressure) that keeps this vital fluid moving comes from the pumping action of the heart. In addition to this, a complex system of nerve signals, hormones, and other elements, regulate the flow by widening or constricting small muscular blood vessels called arterioles.

The heart is nourished by the blood which passes through it own coronary arteries – the heart's main weak spot. Should they become narrowed through cardiovascular disease, the amount of blood able to pass through the heart is reduced. The more heart muscle that is affected by this lack of blood, the less efficient the heart becomes. Sadly, heart disease is the number one cause of death in the Western world.

Except in advanced cases of heart disease, massage with appropriate essential oils is a supremely effective way of improving the circulation. It also stimulates the elimination of excess fluids and tissue wastes via the lymphatic system – a vast network of vessels throughout the body (similar to blood vessels) which transport a watery fluid known as lymph. Unlike the circulatory system, which is controlled by the pumping action of the heart, the lymphatic system has to rely on the normal contractions and relaxation of the muscles through everyday movement, and the force of gravity, to keep the lymph flowing.

Complaints such as arthritis, cellulite, high blood pressure and even depression have been linked with poor lymphatic drainage. As well as regular self-massage (page 21) with essential oils, you can improve your circulation and general well-being by taking adequate exercise, and also dry skin-brushing (page 20) assists lymphatic drainage.

Of course, serious circulatory ailments such as heart disease and chronic high blood pressure must be treated under medical supervision. This chapter continues with some aromatic treatments for minor circulatory ailments which respond well to self-help procedures.

Cellulite

Many doctors insist that cellulite is simply fat, even though it develops in slender bodies as well. Health and beauty experts, on the other hand, believe the dimpled 'orange peel' flesh that appears mostly on the thighs, buttocks and upper arms, is caused by a build-up of tissue wastes.

Below the outer (epidermis) and dermal layers of the skin lies a layer of fat. There is more of this fat in the female body, hence the reason why cellulite is more likely to develop in women. The fat cells are kept apart by connective tissue. Certain conditions cause the connective tissue to degenerate, pushing the fat cells together in an irregular shape and closer to the surface of the skin. Cellulite differs from ordinary fat because it is surrounded by pockets of fluid, resulting from diminished lymphatic drainage from the area.

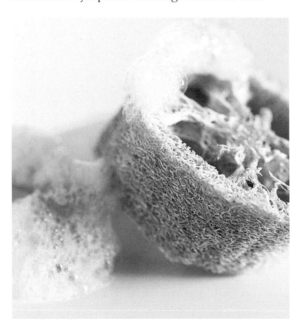

A friction rub improves circulation

It is impossible to eradicate excessive cellulite without resorting to cosmetic surgery (certainly not recommended in this book!). Nevertheless, the treatment strategy outlined here will improve the appearance of 'orange peel' skin. More importantly, it will benefit your health in general.

Take regular exercise (for example, walking or swimming). To protect against 'internal pollution', eat a low fat, high fibre diet with wholegrains, fresh fruit and vegetables (preferably organic). Chemical food additives and excessive consumption of salt, caffeine and alcohol are thought to contribute to the condition. Drink lots of bottled water to keep your system clear, including a couple of mugfuls of warm water every day after breakfast to stimulate the bowels. And, of course, body brushing (see page 20) is an essential part of any anti-cellulite regime. You might also like to incorporate the following aromatic treatments, based on essential oils which are believed to assist lymphatic drainage.

◊ Anti-Cellulite Body Scrub

This scrub is an excellent way of improving skin tone and improving the appearance of orange peel thighs, buttocks and upper arms. Carry out the treatment once or twice a week, as an adjunct to body brushing for the rest of the week. By whisking away the dead skin cells this scrub also makes the skin more receptive to the Anti-Cellulite Body Oil, which should be massaged into the skin immediately afterwards.

3 tablespoons ground oatmeal
4 drops juniper berry essential oil
2 tablespoons freshly-squeezed lemon juice

Mix the ingredients together to form a thick paste. This is a messy treatment, so apply while standing in the bath or shower cubicle. Using circular movements, massage into your skin for at least three minutes before taking a shower.

◖ Anti-Cellulite Body Oil

25ml sweet almond oil
5 drops cypress essential oil
2 drops geranium essential oil
5 drops rosemary essential oil

Massage into the affected areas. Use three times a week in conjunction with skin-brushing or the anti-cellulite body scrub.

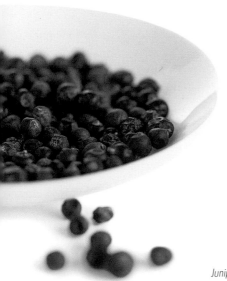

Juniper berry oil for the Anti-Cellulite Body Scrub

If you are prone to cold hands and feet, have poor muscle tone and feel tired most of the day, a daily friction rub is highly recommended. They are energizing, impart a sense of well-being, improve circulation and give the skin a healthy glow. The first recipe is a water-based friction rub if you do not wish to apply oil to the skin, and the second is a traditional massage oil blend.

◖ Water-Based Friction Rub Oil

100ml distilled water
3 teaspoons cider vinegar
1 drop ginger essential oil
1 drop geranium essential oil
1 drop rosemary essential oil

Put the cider vinegar into a dark glass bottle, add the essential oils and shake well. Add the distilled water and shake again. Shake before each use. Apply immediately after your morning shower.

◖ Invigorating Massage Oil

25ml sweet almond oil
1 drop ginger essential oil
1 drop lemongrass essential oil
2 drops rosemary essential oil
2 drops geranium essential oil
2 drops lavender essential oil

Put the sweet almond oil into a dark glass bottle, add the essential oils and shake well. Use as described above.

Varicose Veins & Haemorrhoids

Varicose veins are swollen, knotted blood vessels, usually found in the calves. When they develop in the rectum they are known as haemorrhoids or piles, resulting in itching and sometimes bleeding. This condition generally has multiple causes. A hereditary weakness is usually exacerbated by long periods of standing or increased abdominal pressure through pregnancy or heavy lifting. With haemorrhoids in particular, the varicosity is often associated with chronic constipation (see page 71), which leads to straining during bowel movement.

The best exercises are walking and swimming. Yoga is beneficial too, especially inverted postures. Alternatively rest with your feet higher than your head for 10 to 15 minutes every day.

In order to strengthen the veins, nutritionists recommend eating foods rich in bioflavonoids, particularly blueberries, cherries and other blue and red-coloured berries. When these are out of season, you could supplement your diet with rutin which is rich in bioflavonoids, found naturally in buckwheat and in the pith of citrus fruits. Together with vitamin C (2 x 500mg daily), rutin will help to relieve pain and swelling.

IMPORTANT: Home aromatherapy and herbal treatments aim to reduce pain and inflammation. Where there is bleeding or ulceration, it is essential to seek urgent medical advice.

Bioflavonoids are found in the pith of citrus fruits

Ointment for Varicose Veins and Haemorrhoids

30g unperfumed skin cream
  (available from pharmacies)
1 teaspoon calendula tincture
1 teaspoon hypericum tincture
5 drops frankincense (or cypress) essential oil

Put the skin cream into a little glass pot. Add the tinctures and essential oil and stir until thoroughly mixed. Apply two or three times daily.

For haemorrhoids, apply with a gauze dressing, leaving this in place if possible, and repeat several times daily or whenever painful.

Alternate Hot and Cold Sitz Baths for Haemorrhoids

This bath creates a kind of pumping action which stimulates venous and lymphatic drainage, thus reducing pain and inflammation.

2 bowls large enough to sit in
Comfortably hot water, enough to half-fill a bowl
Tolerably cold water, enough to half-fill a bowl

Sit in the hot bath, and put your feet in the cold bath. Stay there for three minutes, then change position. Sit in the cold bath with your feet in the hot water, and stay there for 30 to 60 seconds. Repeat the cycle two or three times, concluding with the pelvic area immersed in the cold water. Carry out once or twice a day for several days as necessary.

Chilblains

Chilblains occur due to inflammation of the skin. The affected area (usually the fingers, toes, ears or nose) becomes swollen and itchy, sometimes leading to ulceration. The condition is caused by exposure to cold, coupled with poor circulation. Plenty of exercise and regular aromatherapy massage are excellent ways to improve circulation and prevent chilblains. To treat the condition, try the following aromatic remedies.

◍ Chilblain Ointment

200g unperfumed skin cream
  (available from pharmacies)
3 drops sweet marjoram essential oil
3 drops Roman chamomile essential oil
3 drops lemon essential oil

Put the skin cream into a little cosmetic pot, then stir in the essential oils until thoroughly mixed. Apply two or three times a day.

◍ Hand or Foot Bath

6ltrs (3pts) comfortably hot water
1 tablespoon cider vinegar
1 drop black pepper
2 drops rosemary essential oil
2 drops coriander essential oil

Mix the cider vinegar and essential oils together. Pour the hot water into a basin, then add the aromatic vinegar and swish around to disperse. Soak hands or feet for 15 minutes, once or twice daily.

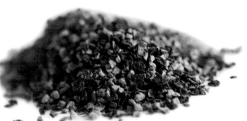

Black pepper improves circulation

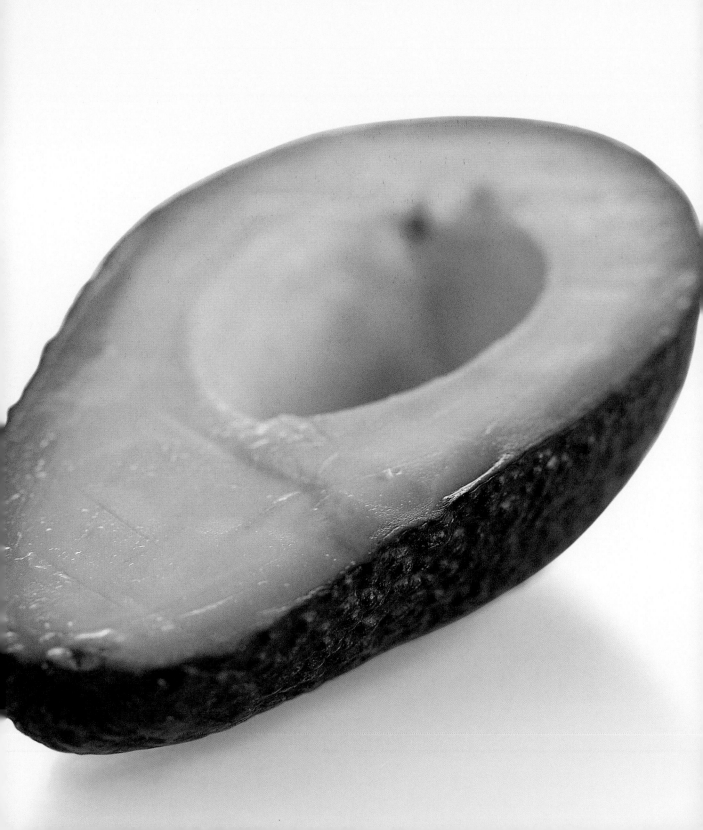

The Digestive System

Eating habits apart, the functioning of the digestive system is closely related to our emotional state. Almost everyone has experienced a 'gut reaction' to a powerful emotion such as fear, anger or anxiety. This may have caused a momentary tightening of the abdomen, or a fluttering sensation in the solar plexus. Prolonged distress, however, can lead to disturbances ranging from diminished appetite, constipation and heartburn, to diarrhoea, nausea or, more seriously, a gastric ulcer.

To help prevent such problems, seek to reduce the stress in your life – for example, by taking up yoga or simply using a relaxation tape.

If you lead a sedentary life and consequently suffer from constipation, a brisk 30-minute walk every day should get things moving again! As well as ensuring that you have enough fibre in your diet (mainly from wholegrains, fresh fruits and vegetables), drink a couple of mugfuls of warm bottled water before or after breakfast as it is an effective method of stimulating sluggish bowels. Laxatives should be avoided if possible (even 'natural' ones from the health store) as these can cause dependency – the bowels ceasing to function properly without them. Chronic constipation should be investigated by a doctor, perhaps followed by treatment from a professional medical herbalist or nutritional therapist.

Regarding nutrition in general, arguments abound as to what constitutes a well-balanced diet. One minute we are told to avoid all animal fat because it is bad for the heart, and to eat polyunsaturated vegetable oils and soft margarines instead. The next moment we are told that, far from being healthy alternatives, many highly-refined vegetable oils and margarines actually contribute to heart disease and poor health in general. While some nutritionists advocate drinking up to three glasses of red wine a day to promote good digestion and a healthy heart, others regard any amount of alcohol as poison! And so it goes on.

Since the experts cannot agree, it is safe to conclude that there is no single ideal diet suitable for everyone. We are each very different, with varying physical needs and personal philosophies. Some people, for example, are drawn to the vegetarian or vegan ideal. For others, the Hay diet is the answer (whereby starches and proteins are not eaten at the same meal). Certainly, if digestive problems persist, despite eating what you consider to be a sensible diet, it is advisable to consult a health professional.

Fresh fruit aids digestion

Before looking at the following treatments, it is important to mention that the external use of essential oils has limited value with regards to the direct treatment of digestive problems such as constipation and diarrhoea. However, if the problem is stress-related, regular aromatherapy massage (ideally treatment by a professional), along with aromatherapy techniques for mood-enhancement (see Mind and Spirit, page 92) can help indirectly by calming a frantic nervous system and lifting the spirits.

Below are some home treatments for the few digestive ailments (also gum problems) that can be helped directly by the use of essential oils. Where appropriate, gentle aromatic herbal remedies are included in the treatment strategies, as these often work more effectively in combination with aromatherapy.

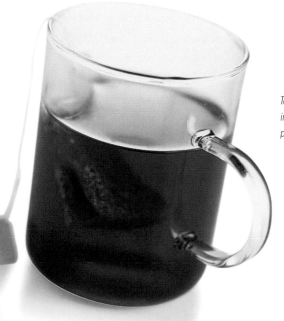

To relieve indigestion try peppermint tea

Indigestion (Heartburn)

Indigestion is a general term for discomfort such as heartburn (which is caused by acid from the stomach travelling up the food pipe), nausea, pain, wind or bloaing in the abdomen brought on by eating. Common causes of indigestion are too much rich food and drink, irregular meals, eating too quickly, arguments at meal times (a common cause!), incompatible food combinations (for example bread with citrus fruits can upset some people), and nervous tension. As well as cutting out the foods you know can bring on indigestion, eat small, regular meals and avoid eating late at night. Above all, eat in convivial surroundings – and allow time to enjoy your food!

Peppermint tea is a wonderful remedy for all kinds of indigestion, and is available in tea bag form from supermarkets. If you dislike the taste of peppermint, try fennel, lemon balm or chamomile (see also the herb tea blends given on page 75). The simplest and most effective aromatherapy treatment is to put two to three drops of peppermint oil (or indeed, any other oil recommended for indigestion) onto a tissue and inhale deeply every couple of minutes until you experience relief. As a preventative remedy, try one of the following vaporizing blends which can be enjoyed at mealtimes. If you dislike any of the essential oils given in the recipe, refer to the Quick Guide to Essential Oils (see page 134) where you will find a number of alternatives.

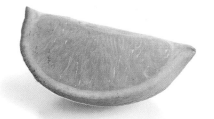

Try lime essential oil in a vaporizer to promote good digestion

◍ Bon Appetit! Vaporizing Blends

RECIPE 1

1 drop cardamom essential oil

3 drops lemon essential oil

2 drops neroli (or petitgrain) essential oil

RECIPE 2

2 drops lemon essential oil

1 drop lime essential oil

4 drops bergamot essential oil

RECIPE 3

1 drop peppermint essential oil

1 drop rosemary essential oil

1 drop clary sage essential oil

3 drops lemon essential oil

Add the essential oils to the water-filled dish of the vaporizer, then light the candle. For electric vaporizers, follow the manufacturer's instructions.

Nausea (Motion Sickness)

The causes of nausea include stress, constipation, faulty diet, overeating, mild food poisoning, indigestion, pregnancy and motion sickness. Fresh air tends to alleviate all nausea. Persistent nausea with no apparent cause should be investigated by a doctor.

Many herbal remedies and their essential oils can quell nausea – but only if the aroma and taste are found agreeable. If not, the herb or oil is more likely to cause vomiting! Of the herb teas, that help alleviate nausea, lemon balm, peppermint and chamomile are the easiest to obtain from supermarkets. For motion and pregnancy sickness, many people experience relief from sucking a little crystallized stem ginger (available from good supermarkets and grocers). Travel sickness tablets containing ginger are available from health stores.

If you have a garden and are able to grow the beautiful aromatic herb angelica (*Angelica archangelica*) the sharp-tasting leaves are renowned for their ability to quell nausea. Simply tear off a fresh leaf and chew.

The most effective aromatherapy treatment for nausea (including motion sickness) is to put a few drops of an essential oil such as peppermint (or any other oil recommended for nausea, see page 136) on a tissue and inhale deeply every few minutes until you experience relief.

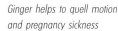

Ginger helps to quell motion and pregnancy sickness

Gingivitis

Gingivitis is inflammation of the gums, which then tend to bleed when the teeth are brushed. The condition is caused by poor oral hygiene and a diet high in sugar and processed foods. If left untreated, it may develop into severe gum disease (pyorrhoea) and tooth loss. Gentle, regular and effective brushing and flossing are essential. But do ensure that your toothbrush is neither too hard or too soft (check with your dentist).

Use a natural toothpaste containing plant extracts such as myrrh, aloe vera, fennel, arnica or calendula. Visit your dentist regularly (preferably one who practises holistic dentistry). You will also find the following antiseptic, gum-strengthening mouthwash beneficial.

◖ Mouthwash for Bleeding Gums

½ teaspoon calendula tincture
1 drop tea tree essential oil
1 teacup lukewarm water

Put the calendula tincture into the cup, then add the essential oil, and top up with warm water. After brushing your teeth, use the mixture to rinse out your mouth several times.

Mouth Ulcers

An ulcerous sore (or a cluster of sores) inside the cheek, lips or the gum. Sometimes they are initiated by inadvertently biting the inside of the mouth or by irritation from a denture. Quite often they are indicative of a run-down condition resulting from stress, illness or antibiotic treatment. If you have mouth ulcers for more than a month, consult your doctor as the condition can be symptomatic of a more serious ailment such as ulcerative colitis or coliac disease.

Generally, it can be beneficial to supplement your daily diet with a good multivitamin and mineral formula, along with 2 x 500mg vitamin C. Avoid vinegar, lemons, pickles, mustard and salted snacks as these are likely to cause pain when they come into contact with the sore. If your mouth is sore enough to stop you from eating, drink freshly squeezed organic vegetable or fruit juices. Additionally, try the following aromatic remedy.

◖ Treatment for Mouth Ulcers

½ teaspoon calendula tincture
1 drop myrrh essential oil
1 teacup lukewarm water

Put the calendula tincture into a cup, add the essential oil, then top up with warm water. If used as a mouthwash three or four times daily, the ulcers should heal within five days.

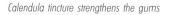

Calendula tincture strengthens the gums

Irritable Bowel Syndrome (IBS)

The characteristics of IBS are persistent and recurrent abdominal pains, usually gripping but sometimes with sharp or cutting episodes, bloating, irregular bowel habits with diarrhoea or constipation, flatulence and associated nausea, and lethargy. Food sensitivities are also implicated. Common triggers commonly include milk products, wheat, meat and sugar. Ideally, consult a qualified nutritionist who will help you to identify the food culprits.

There is no doubt that prolonged stress is a principal factor in IBS. Therefore, it is certainly worth considering taking up yoga, meditation, t'ai chi or some other form of stress relief, as these really can help reduce symptoms (see also the Mind recipes on page 92). Hypnotherapy has helped many IBS sufferers who have exhausted other options, but it is essential to see a registered therapist in order to learn the techniques.

As well as using aromatherapy to reduce stress, studies have shown that peppermint oil can be used as a specific remedy. Taken internally in the form of peppermint oil capsules, it has a strong antispasmodic action and will act to relieve, although probably not cure, IBS. Peppermint oil capsules are available from health stores (take as directed on the label). If peppermint oil capsules are unavailable, try one of the following herbal teas.

Rosemary calms IBS

Antispasmodic Teas for IBS

RECIPE 1
300ml boiling water
2 teaspoons dried chamomile flowers
1 teaspoon dried rosemary
1 teaspoon dried sage

RECIPE 2
2 teaspoons dried peppermint
1 teaspoon dried lemon balm
1 teaspoon dried lavender flowers

RECIPE 3
2 teaspoons dried spearmint
1 teaspoon dried sweet marjoram
1 teaspoon dried sage

Put the herbs into a teapot or heatproof jug, then add the boiling water. Allow to infuse for 10 to 15 minutes. To help alleviate the abdominal pain and bloating caused by IBS, drink a teacupful every two hours.

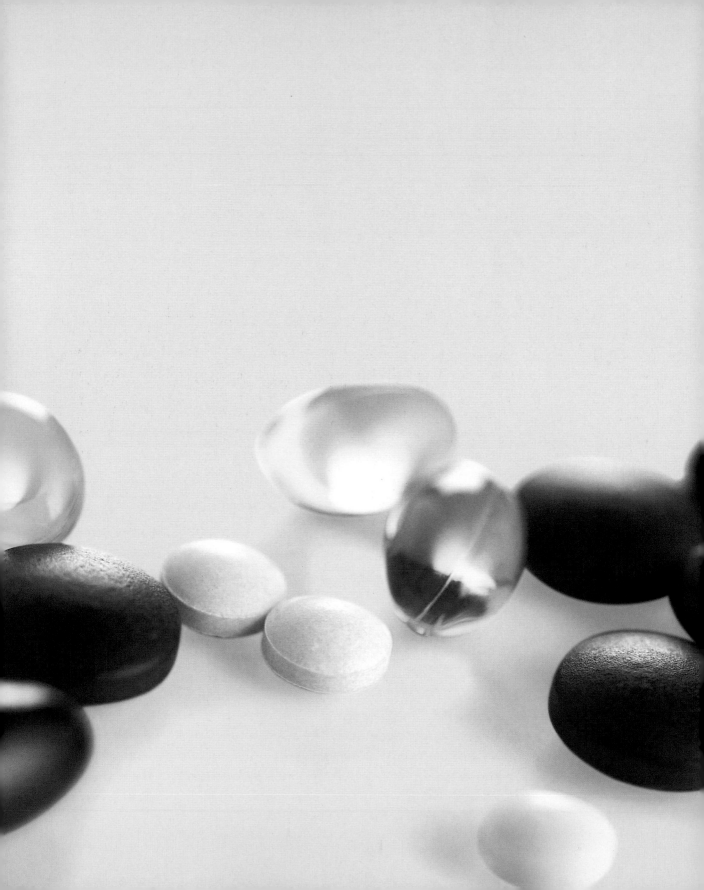

Muscles and Joints

While the skeleton gives form and support to the body, the muscles are composed of flexible tissue and are concerned with movement. When our muscles and joints are supple and mobile, we radiate vitality and are more resilient to the stresses and strains of life.

It is often reported that more people take time off work as a result of back problems than for any other condition. This may be caused or aggravated by many factors, including poor posture, prolonged sitting, incorrect lifting of heavy loads, or prolonged emotional stress. Quite a common problem affecting the spine is the so-called slipped disc. Between each pair of vertebrae are cartilage discs containing a resilient, jelly-like substance. The purpose of these discs is to act as shock absorbers, thus preventing the vertebrae from grinding together whenever we move. However, a severe jolt caused by a fall, for example, can rupture the disc's tough envelope, permitting the enclosed jelly to ooze out. This material then presses on a nerve which results in excruciating pain. This is because the irritated nerve causes the surrounding muscle to go into spasm. A slipped disc is best dealt with by an osteopath or chiropractor, though sea-salt baths and aromatherapy massage can ease discomfort during the recovery period.

Apart from those aches and pains associated with strenuous activity and general wear and tear, the most common problems affecting muscular and skeletal system are arthritis and rheumatism. Many different forms are recognized by doctors, including bursitis, gout, osteoarthritis and rheumatic arthritis. All are painful and restrict movement. There may also be inflammation and swelling, calcification of the joints, and loss of synovial fluid, which lubricates joints.

The conventional medical approach is to prescribe anti-inflammatory drugs and sometimes corticosteroids, all of which can have unpleasant side-effects. Surgery, such as hip replacement, may also play a part. Yet there are many recorded cases of people who have used natural therapies such as acupuncture, massage, herbal medicine, homoeopathy and dietary reform to greatly reduce pain and increase mobility. If you suffer from any diseases of the muscular and skeletal system, it is well worth consulting a qualified complementary health practitioner who will be able to devise a treatment strategy geared to your specific needs.

Arthritis and Rheumatism

While aromatherapy can help reduce pain and inflammation, it cannot tackle the underlying cause of the condition – be it faulty nutrition, prolonged physical and emotional stress, heredity or a combination of factors. In addition to the advice given above, gentle exercise such as walking or swimming will improve mobility in the joints. Try to reduce the level of stress in your life, perhaps by taking up meditation or listening to a relaxation and visualization tape.

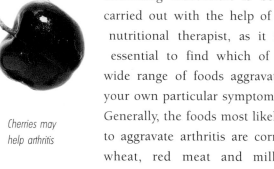

The dietary approach to alleviating discomfort is best carried out with the help of a nutritional therapist, as it is essential to find which of a wide range of foods aggravate your own particular symptoms. Generally, the foods most likely to aggravate arthritis are corn, wheat, red meat and milk. Foods that may help ease discomfort are cherries, and oily fish such as salmon, mackerel, tuna or sardine. They are rich in omega-3 fatty acids which can help maintain and improve the suppleness of the joints. Fish oil supplements are available from pharmacies and health stores (take as directed). If you are vegetarian, the finest nutritional supplement for easing pain and inflammation is evening primrose oil (3 x 500mg daily). The anti-inflammatory herbal remedy meadowsweet is also worth trying.

Cherries may help arthritis

AROMATHERAPY TREATMENTS

The most effective aromatherapy treatments are baths, massage and compresses. The body responds best if it does not become too accustomed to a particular essential oil or blend of oils. So it is important to use the following aromatic concentrates in rotation. Apply Recipe 1 for a month, then give your body a rest from all essential oils for a week. Resume treatment with Recipe 2 for the next month, then give your body another week's break, before continuing with Recipe 1 for a third month, and so on.

RECIPE 1
◊ Aromatic Concentrate for Arthritic and Rheumatic Pain

15 drops carrot seed essential oil
10 drops Atlas cedarwood essential oil
10 drops coriander essential oil
10 drops lemon essential oil

Put the essential oils into a little dark glass bottle and shake well.

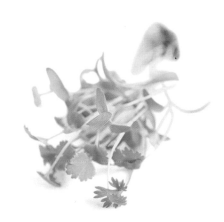

Coriander oil is captured from the seed of the herb

RECIPE 2

🌢 Aromatic Concentrate for Arthritic and Rheumatic Pain

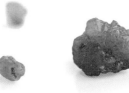

Ease the pain of arthritis with a blend including frankincense

10 drops juniper berry essential oil
15 drops lavender essential oil
10 drops rosemary essential oil
10 drops frankincense essential oil

Put the essential oils into a little dark glass bottle and shake well.

METHODS OF USE

Aromatic Salt Bath (comfortably hot): *Add 200 to 300g Dead Sea Mineral Salts to the bath while the water is still running. After the bath has been filled, add eight drops of essential oil concentrate and swish around to disperse. Take an aromatic bath daily, or at least three times weekly.*

Massage Oil: *Add 12 drops of concentrate to 25ml sweet almond oil and shake well. Massage into the affected parts two or three times daily, including after an aromatic bath.*

CAUTION: Never massage inflamed and swollen joints as this will increase heat in the tissues, causing further discomfort. Instead, apply a cold compress. With rheumatoid arthritis, for example, inflammation comes and goes, so massage over affected parts is fine between flare-ups, and may even reduce the frequency of attacks.

Compress (hot or cold): *If there is any swelling or inflammation around the joint (the skin over an inflamed joint usually feels quite hot), use a cold compress. For dull aches and pains, use a hot compress. Add five drops of concentrate to a bowl containing 600ml (1pt) of water. Soak a piece of clean, folded cotton fabric in the water, wring out the excess and apply to the affected area. As soon as it warms (or cools if using a hot application) to body temperature, re-apply. Repeat once or twice more in succession. Compresses may be applied two or three times daily, or as required.*

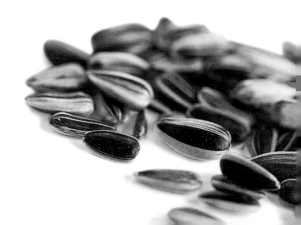

Muscular Aches and Pains

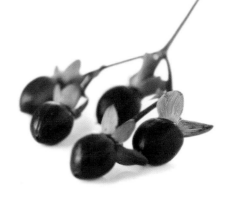

Hypericum berries

Apart from discomfort caused by over-exertion – say, while digging the garden or playing a hectic sport – chronic muscular aches and stiffness may be related to an arthritic or rheumatic complaint, or it may be stress-related. If caused by a recent injury, the pain will be sharp or searing, in which case, a cold compress with German chamomile (five drops in 600ml water) would be most helpful. Old injuries and muscular tension manifest as a dull ache, and so benefit from hot baths and massage.

◔ Aromatic Vinegar Bath for Sore Muscles

Cider vinegar, as well as being beneficial to the skin, is an age-old remedy for aching muscles. In this recipe its soothing properties are increased with the addition of muscle-relaxant essential oils.

6 tablespoons cider vinegar
2 drops rosemary essential oil
2 drops black pepper essential oil
2 drops sweet marjoram essential oil
2 drops lavender essential oil

Add the vinegar and essential oils to the bath after it has been filled, then swish around to disperse.

◔ Hercules Muscle Oil

15ml macerated hypericum oil (or use virgin olive oil)
20ml sunflower seed oil
6 drops sweet marjoram essential oil

3 drops coriander essential oil
3 drops clary sage essential oil
4 drops grapefruit essential oil

Funnel the hypericum and sunflower seed oils into a dark glass bottle, add the essential oils and shake well. Massage into the muscles two or three times daily, including immediately after an aromatic bath.

◔ Sampson Muscle Oil

25ml virgin olive oil
4 drops German chamomile
4 drops rosemary
3 drops lemon

Funnel the olive oil into a dark glass bottle, add the essential oils and shake well. Massage into the muscles two or three times a day, including immediately after an aromatic bath.

Muscles and Joints First Aid

SPRAIN

A sprain occurs at a joint such as a wrist or ankle when the ligaments and tissues around it are wrenched or torn. The symptoms are pain and tenderness around the joint, often followed by swelling and bruising. After treating the sprain with essential oils, rest the injured limb and raise it above the level of your head to prevent accumulation of excess fluids (support with cushions or pillows). Treatment must always begin with a cold or icy compress to reduce pain and swelling. Afterwards, apply the cooling gel to encourage healing of the damaged tissues.

◉ Cold Compress

1pt cold water (preferably with some ice cubes)
4 drops German chamomile (or lavender) essential oil

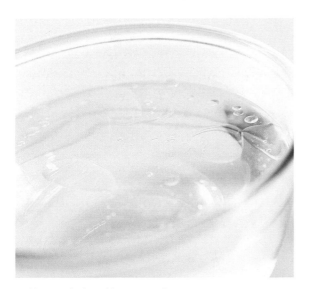

Add essential oil to cold water to make a compress

Pour the water into a bowl, add the essential oil and swish around to disperse. Soak a piece of clean, folded cotton fabric in the water, wring out the excess and apply to the affected part. As soon as it warms to body temperature, re-apply. Repeat two or three times, adding more ice to the water as neccessary.

◉ Cooling Gel for Sprains

25ml aloe vera gel
1 drop peppermint essential oil
2 drops lavender essential oil

Put the aloe vera gel into a little glass pot, add the essential oils and stir well. Apply to the injured area two or three times daily.

STRAIN (MUSCULAR)

A strain occurs when a muscle or group of muscles is overstretched, and possibly torn, by violent or sudden movement – for example back strain as a result of heavy lifting. After treatment with a cold compress to help reduce pain and inflammation, rest is important. If you have strained the muscle of an arm or leg, raise the injured part above the level of your head to prevent accumulation of excess fluids (support with cushions or pillows).

◉ Cold Compress

600ml cold or tepid water
2 drops rosemary essential oil
2 drops lavender essential oil

Pour the water into a bowl, add the essential oil and swish around to disperse. Soak a piece of clean, folded cotton fabric in the water, wring out the excess and apply to the affected part. As soon as it warms to body temperature, re-apply. Repeat two or three times.

⬥ Aromatic Salt Bath

Once the swelling has subsided (after treatment with cold compresses), aromatic salt baths will relax taut muscles and facilitate healing of damaged tissue.

200g Dead Sea Mineral Salts
5 drops rosemary essential oil
2 drops geranium essential oil
1 drop helichrysum (or ginger) essential oil

Add the Dead Sea salts to the bath while the water is still running. After the bath has been filled, add the essential oils and swish around to disperse. Take this aromatic salt bath once a day for about a week.

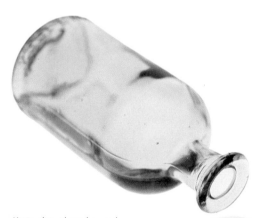

Virgin olive oil can be used in massage blends

CRAMP

An overworked muscle in the foot or leg may suddenly go into spasm causing excruciating pain. The first step in relieving the pain is to stretch the cramped muscle. In many cases, simply walking on the affected limb is enough to release the spasm. If this does not work, however, you will need to flex and massage the affected area.

To relieve cramp in the foot, grasp the toes and gently bend them back towards the body while holding the heel with the other hand. Then stroke the sole of the foot with the heel of your hand or your thumb.

Calf cramps can be eased by flexing the entire foot so that the toes are pointing towards the body and there is a pulling sensation in the affected muscles. Knead the muscles firmly, working from the bottom of the leg up to the knee and back down again.

To relieve hamstring cramp, lie on your back and raise the affected leg with the knee straight and the toes of the foot bent towards the shin bone. Next stroke the back of the thigh towards the buttocks.

Usually there is no need to apply oils to ease cramp. However, if the pain does return, even after you have carried out the above procedures, try one of the following massage blends.

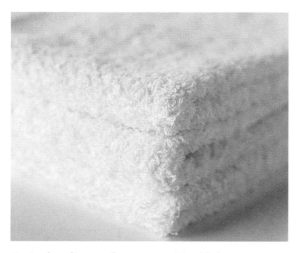

Use towels, cushions or pillows to support injured limbs

RECIPE 4

25ml sweet almond oil

2 drops vetiver essential oil

4 drops lavender essential oil

2 drops grapefruit essential oil

2 drops coriander essential oil

Funnel the vegetable base oil into a dark glass bottle, add the essential oils and shake well. You may prefer to mix a smaller amount of oil for this first-aid procedure, enough for a single treatment. If so, mix the oils together in a small dish or a saucer and reduce the quantity by half.

◆ Massage Oils for Muscular Cramp

RECIPE 1

25ml virgin olive oil

3 drops Roman chamomile essential oil

5 drops lavender essential oil

3 drops sweet marjoram essential oil

RECIPE 2

25ml sweet almond oil

4 drops cypress essential oil

2 drops black pepper essential oil

4 drops rosemary essential oil

RECIPE 3

25ml macerated hypericum oil

2 drops rosemary essential oil

2 drops lavender essential oil

1 drop German chamomile essential oil

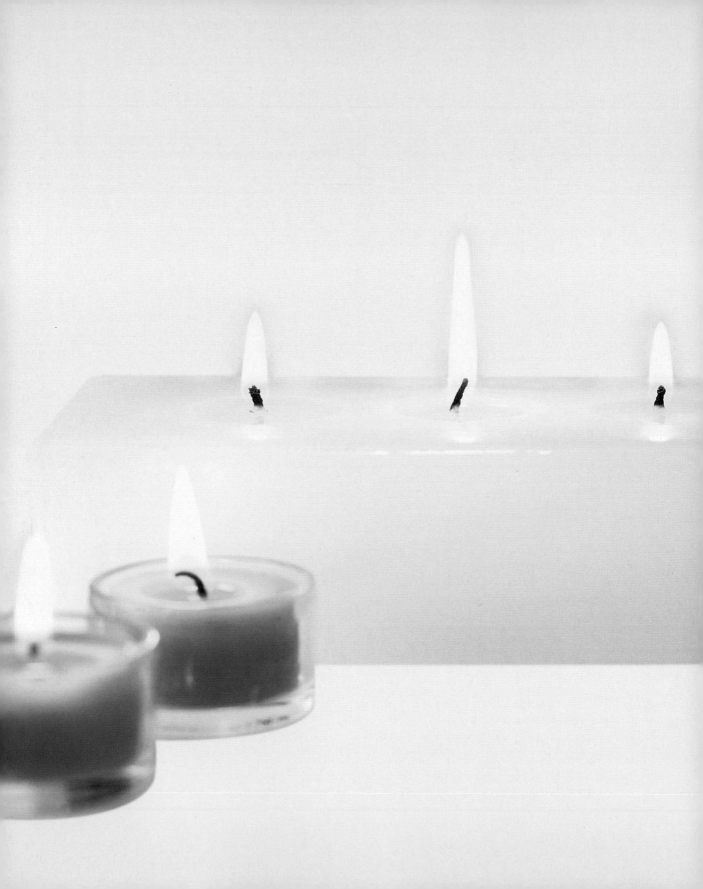

Women's Health

Aromatherapy is especially beneficial for women's health. Apart from the mood-enhancing and stress-reducing properties of essential oils (see the Mind and Spirit section, page 92), they can exert a specific effect on the female reproductive system. It has been confirmed by pharmacognosists (those who study the chemical composition of plants) and pharmacologists (those who study the effects of substances on the human physio-logical processes) that a number of plants such as hops, fennel and sage contain oestrogen-like substances (phyto-oestrogens), which have been shown to regulate the menstrual cycle and minimize menopausal symptoms like hot flushes and mood swings. The essential oils of such plants are thought to retain these hormone-like compounds.

Certain foods also contain phyto-oestrogens and are highly beneficial to women's health (they are nutritious for men too). Unlike synthetic oestrogens, whose chemistry differs and which must be cautiously administered to reduce side effects, phyto-oestrogens found in certain foods and herbs are totally compatible with the human body and help protect against many conditions affecting the female reproductive system.

According to Herman Aldercreutz, nutritional chemist at the University of Helsinki, and others, the best protective foodstuffs are tofu (soya bean curd), miso (fermented soya paste), rye bread, green lentils, pomegranates and French beans. Other foods which contain hormone-affecting prop-erties are sprouted seeds and grains (especially alfalfa), celery, papaya, bananas, figs, dates, apples, grapes, cherries, citrus fruits, anise, avocado, liquorice, edible seaweed products, garlic, beetroot, potatoes, aubergine and parsley.

So, if you are experiencing distressing menopausal symptoms, suffer from PMS or other menstrual problems, it is certainly worth looking at your diet. Should symptoms be particularly troublesome, aromatherapy is a marvellous supportive measure.

IMPORTANT: The aromatherapy formulations given below may not be right for every woman. Some of the recipes will almost certainly need to be adjusted to suit individual aroma preferences. If the aroma is disliked, the blend is unlikely to embrace the emotions which play an important role in hormonal balance. To widen your choice of oils for specific ailments, refer to the Quick Guide to Essential Oils (page 134).

*Bananas may help
balance hormones*

Amenorrhoea (loss of periods)

Periods can become irregular, scanty, or cease altogether, for many reasons, including stress, sudden weight loss, anorexia nervosa, over-exercise, thyroid disease, anaemia, and, of course, during pregnancy and breastfeeding. In older women the condition may herald the start of menopause. If your periods stop suddenly for no apparent reason, it is advisable to have a medical check-up to rule out the possibility of a serious underlying health problem.

With regards to exercise, as with most aspects of human health, going to the extreme can be dangerous. Prolonged strenuous training produces rapid changes in hormone levels. It can reduce the amount of oestrogen to such an extent that periods cease altogether. If the body fat stores diminish too much, young women become vulnerable to some of the problems that can afflict post-menopausal women. So never allow yourself to exercise or under-eat to such a degree that your periods stop. It may temporarily improve your physical performance, but your bones are likely to remain vulnerable to fractures for the rest of your life.

If your life is stressful, practise yoga, t'ai chi or some other system of relaxation and movement. Drink sage tea (available from health stores), a traditional remedy for menstrual problems. A course of professional aromatherapy massage treatments (for example, a full-body massage once a week for a month) will balance your whole system and may well promote normal menstruation. Home aromatherapy treatments may also prove beneficial. However, if there is no sign of improvement after six to eight weeks of regular use of appropriate essential oils, do consult a professional health practitioner.

◆ Essential Oil Concentrate (for promoting menstruation)

15 drops Virginian cedarwood essential oil
6 drops coriander essential oil
10 drops clary sage essential oil
12 drops rose otto essential oil

Put the essential oils into a dark glass bottle and shake well. For the following applications, dispense the concentrate using a pipette or eye dropper (available from pharmacies).

METHODS OF USE

Bath: *Add six drops of the concentrate to your daily bath. Or, take the bath at least three times a week in conjunction with massage and dry inhalations.*

Massage: *25ml sweet almond oil, 10 drops of the concentrate. Massage a little of the oil into your abdomen immediately after your daily bath or shower.*

Dry Inhalation: *Put a few drops of the concentrate (or choose a single essential oil recommended for amenorrhoea) on a tissue and inhale at intervals throughout the day. This supportive treatment should be used in combination with aromatic baths and massage oil.*

Only use rubber-tipped droppers for dispensing diluted oils

Dysmenorrhoea (painful periods)

Period pain is more common in young women and tends to ease after the age of 25. Persistent or excruciating pain should always be investigated by a doctor, as it may be symptomatic of a serious gynaecological disorder. This could perhaps be followed by professional treatment from a medical herbalist or homoeopath. For home treatment, try raspberry leaf tea (available from health stores) or the tea suggested below. The following aromatherapy treatments will also help.

◗ Essential Oil Concentrate for Period Pain

10 drops rosemary essential oil
15 drops lavender essential oil
15 drops sweet marjoram essential oil

Put the essential oils into a dark glass bottle and shake well. For the following applications, dispense using a pipette or eye dropper (available from pharmacies).

METHODS OF USE
Bath: *Add eight drops of the concentrate to your bath.*

Massage: *25ml sweet almond oil, 10 drops of the concentrate. Immediately after your bath or shower, smooth a little of the oil into your abdomen, then do feather-light stroking with your fingertips downwards over the abdomen for about five minutes.*

This movement will help alleviate pain and congestion. Ideally, ask a friend or partner to do the feather-light massage for you. This will enable you to lie back and relax with your knees bent (supported by cushions) to ease any pain in the lumbar region.

Hot Compress: *For some women, this method is the most effective. Put about a litre of comfortably hot water in a basin, then add five drops of the concentrate and swish around to disperse. Soak a hand towel in the water, wring out the excess and apply to the abdomen. Cover the compress with a dry, folded towel (or use a sheet of cling film) to conserve the heat. As soon as the compress cools to body temperature, reapply if necessary.*

◗ Melissa Herb Tea for Painful Periods

(using fresh herbs)
15g lemon balm leaves
10g lavender flowers
15g sweet marjoram
600ml (1pt) boiling water.

Put the herbs into a teapot, add the boiling water and allow to steep for 15 minutes. The tea may be taken hot or cold, sweetened with a little honey if desired. Dosage is one teacupful three times daily.

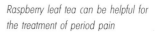

Raspberry leaf tea can be helpful for the treatment of period pain

Menorrhagia (heavy periods)

Periods often become heavier as women approach menopause, but can also indicate a hormonal imbalance, endometriosis, pelvic infection and fibroids in the womb. For heavy bleeding with no known reason, it is essential to consult your doctor.

For home treatment, drink a teacupful of sage tea (available from health stores) three times a day for a week before the expected date of your period.

◆ Essential Oil Concentrate for Heavy Periods

15 drops frankincense essential oil
10 drops cypress essential oil
8 drops geranium essential oil
12 drops lemon essential oil

Put the essential oils into a dark glass bottle and shake well. For the following applications, dispense using a pipette or eye dropper (available from pharmacies).

METHODS OF USE

Bath: *Add eight drops of the concentrate to your daily bath, beginning a week to 10 days before the expected date of your period.*

Massage: *25ml sweet almond oil, 10 drops of the concentrate. Immediately after your bath or shower, smooth a little of the oil into your abdomen and lower back. Begin the treatment a week to 10 days prior to the expected date of your period.*

To avoid morning sickness eat a ginger biscuit

Pregnancy Sickness

Nausea is common in early pregnancy. While it is more likely to occur first thing in the morning, some women feel nauseous at other times of the day as well. The possible causes include changing hormone levels and low blood sugar.

Avoid large, heavy or rich meals and eat smaller portions of plain foods such as boiled rice, steamed or stir-fried vegetables, steamed or poached fish. Ginger is one of the finest natural remedies for nausea. Before getting up in the morning, eat a plain ginger biscuit and during the day drink ginger tea. Add ¼ teaspoon of ground ginger to a mugful of hot water, sweeten with honey and sip. Taking a multivitamin and mineral supplement formulated for pregnancy may also help.

A number of essential oils are recommended for nausea, but of course the aroma must be liked; otherwise it may actually cause vomiting! Choose from the following: lavender, ginger, peppermint, rose otto, cardamom, coriander and Roman chamomile. Put a few drops on a tissue and inhale as required.

NB: Although some of these oils are cited as being unsuitable for use during pregnancy (see page 110), they are perfectly safe for dry inhalation. Cautions generally allude to applications to the skin and internal dosage.

PMS (Premenstrual Syndrome)

This condition was previously called PMT (premenstrual tension); however, 'syndrome' is a more appropriate term because tension is but one of many other symptoms which may be experienced. PMS can begin any time from two days to two weeks prior to menstruation. Symptoms may include fluid retention, breast tenderness, headaches, nausea, anxiety, depression, irritability, sleep disturbances, food cravings and other disturbances. Mercifully, very few women suffer all these symptoms, but all women experience some degree of pre-menstrual change.

As well as taking care of your diet (as explained at the beginning of this chapter) it may be necessary to reduce stress. Consider taking up yoga, t'ai chi or some other system of relaxation and gentle movement (see also page 93). One of the most effective herbal remedies for PMS is *Vitex agnus-castus* or chaste tree berry. Alternatively, you may find evening primrose oil beneficial (dosage 2 x 500mg daily), especially if symptoms include breast tenderness. Both remedies are widely available from pharmacies and health stores. The following aromatherapy treatments can be used as a supportive measure.

◈ Essential Oil Concentrate for PMS

As well as helping to reduce stress and anxiety, the essential oils chosen for this concentrate will deal with other common symptoms of PMS such as headaches, insomnia and fluid retention.

8 drops Roman chamomile essential oil
12 drops lavender essential oil
8 drops clary sage essential oil
8 drops juniper berry essential oil
12 drops mandarin essential oil

Put the essential oils into a dark glass bottle and shake well. For the following applications, dispense using a pipette or eye dropper (available from pharmacies).

METHODS OF USE

Bath: *Add six drops of the concentrate to your daily bath, beginning seven to 10 days before the expected date of your period.*

Massage: *50ml sweet almond oil, 15 to 20 drops of the concentrate. Immediately after your bath or shower, massage the oil into your body. Begin the treatment seven to 10 days prior to the date of your period.*

Dry Inhalation: *Whenever you feel emotional upset during the day, try this method. Put a few drops of the concentrate on a tissue and inhale at intervals. Alternatively, use a single essential oil which makes you feel relaxed and uplifted. A good choice might be rose otto, bergamot, lavender, ylang-ylang or neroli. To help you sleep at night, put a few drops of lavender, Roman chamomile, clary sage or sandalwood on a cotton handkerchief, then place it under your pillow slip.*

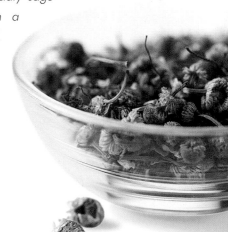

Chamomile alleviates the symptoms of PMS

Menopausal Problems

The menopause heralds the end of menstruation, usually around the age of 45 to 55. While some women sail through the menopause with little discomfort, others may experience symptoms such as hot flushes and night sweats, vaginal dryness and mood swings. Some women suffer from aches and pains, irritability, depression, palpitations, loss of libido, headaches and fatigue.

If you would prefer to avoid HRT and its potential side effects, begin by taking care of your diet (as explained at the beginning of this chapter). It may also help to supplement your diet with 4 x 500mg capsules of evening primrose oil a day to help maintain hormone balance. Excellent nutrition should be combined with weight-bearing exercise such as a 30-minute walk every day. This kind of exercise helps to develop strong bones, thus protecting against osteoporosis which can occur in later life.

If you are experiencing hot flushes and night sweats, the most effective herbal remedy is sage tea (available from health stores). Prepare as directed and drink a teacupful at bedtime, and another every afternoon. Sage is very drying, however, so if you also have vaginal dryness, take *Vitex agues-castus* (chaste tree berry) instead.

Aromatherapy can be used as an adjunct to reduce stress and help balance your system (see also page 93). Clary sage oil is regarded as a specific treatment for treating hot flushes and night sweats.

Use a facial mist to cool a hot flush

◆ Aromatic Vinegar Evening Bath

As well as helping to prevent night sweats, this bath will promote restful sleep.

6 tablespoons cider vinegar
5 drops clary sage essential oil
2 drops lavender essential oil

Mix the essential oils with the vinegar, then add to a comfortably warm (but not hot) bath. During hot weather, you may enjoy this in a lukewarm bath. Relax for at least 15 minutes. Afterwards, you might like to apply some Cooling Body Gel.

◆ Cooling Body Gel for Hot Flushes

50ml aloe vera gel
3 drops clary sage essential oil
3 drops lavender essential oil
1 drop peppermint essential oil

Put the aloe vera gel into a glass pot, then stir in the essential oils until thoroughly mixed. As a preventative, smooth into your skin after a morning bath or shower.

◆ Cool Lady Facial Mist

Here is a simple remedy for cooling your face and neck while actually experiencing a hot flush: squeeze a quantity of aloe vera gel into a cosmetic bottle with a fine mist spray. Dilute with an equal amount of distilled water and shake well. Mist your skin as required. Make a fresh batch every two weeks.

Sore or Cracked Nipples

This problem is common in breastfeeding mothers in the first weeks before their nipples have 'hardened' to the effects of continual sucking. To allow time for healing, wear nipple shields (available from pharmacies). These will enable the baby to suck without causing you discomfort. To promote healing, apply one of the following preparations.

IMPORTANT: Wash off all traces of oil or ointment before each feed.

Hypercal Nipple Oil

20ml macerated calendula oil
20ml macerated hypericum oil

Put the oils into a dark glass bottle and shake well. Apply after each feed.

Hypercal Nipple Cream

25g unperfumed skin cream
  (available from pharmacies)
1 teaspoon calendula tincture
1 teaspoon hypericum tincture

Put the skin cream into a little glass pot, stir in the tinctures until thoroughly mixed. Apply after each feed.

*Skin cream to calm
sore nipples*

Breastfeeding

Many mothers worry endlessly and often unnecessarily about the quantity and quality of their milk. If you are a breastfeeding mother and have a good wholefood diet (including drinking plenty of bottled water), are free of major stress, chronic illness and your lifestyle allows for adequate rest, fresh air and exercise, then you should experience few problems. If, however, your baby is constantly fretful or listless and fails to gain a reasonable amount of weight, there may be genuine cause for concern, so do seek professional advice from your doctor or midwife.

Herbal mixtures such as the aromatic tea below, have been used for centuries by nursing mothers to increase milk flow.

Aromatic Seed Infusion for Breastfeeding Mothers

1½ teaspoons fennel seed
½ teaspoon caraway seed
½ teaspoon fenugreek seed
1 ltr (1½pts water)

Put the seeds into a stainless steel saucepan, add the water and bring to the boil. Turn down the heat and simmer for 15 minutes. The dosage is one teacupful three times a day (may be taken hot or cold).

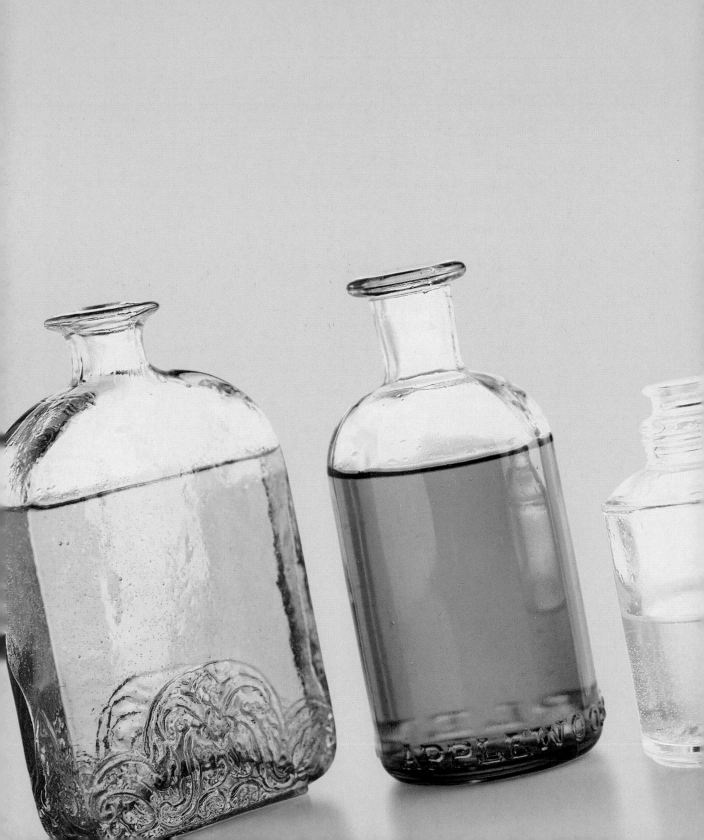

Mind and Spirit

Aromatherapy, in common with all holistic therapies, seeks to nurture the whole person – body, mind and spirit. As well as making good use of nature's essential oils, this is achieved through sound nutrition, adequate exercise, fresh air, moderate amounts of sunlight, sufficient sleep, relaxation and recreation – and, above all, by attending to the needs of the soul.

Although our language offers no absolute definition of 'soul', we might say it encompasses the mental, emotional and spiritual aspects of our being. The mental aspect comprises our intellect, ideas, beliefs and attitudes about the world, often conditioned by the influences of family, schooling and culture. Our emotions, just like the ocean's undercurrents, are the energizing forces which direct and sustain behaviour, adding colour and richness to our daily lives. The spiritual aspect is tied up with our own unique sense of purpose and meaning. Without purpose we become depressed or apathetic; life then appears bleak and meaningless.

Even when we do not follow a conscious spiritual path in terms of a religious faith, we may in fact be nurturing our spiritual self in some other way. It could be through a love of music, painting or some other art form, no matter how humble, or simply through our work, family, relationships, or a love of animals or nature or more actively, perhaps, by working towards the realization of a humanitarian or Green ideal.

Even in cases where the pathological condition has advanced beyond all hope of healing on a physical level, it is still possible to experience healing in a spiritual sense. Indeed, this is the main aim of the hospice movement (which often employs aromatherapists and other holistic therapists), whose task is to enable people to die peacefully in the knowledge that life is not without purpose and meaning. To die peacefully and without fear is the ultimate healing experience.

Stress and the Mind–Body Phenomenon

Since the 1970s, research in the field of psychoneuroimmunology (or PNI) has documented direct links between emotions and physical health, thereby giving scientific credence to what holistic healers have always known: distressing emotions can manifest as physical symptoms, contributing to an overall weakening of the immune system. The effects may be experienced within any part of the body, depending on the individual's innate constitution. For example, there may be raised blood pressure, allergies, skin eruptions, a susceptibility to every passing infection, or something more serious. Emotional disharmony may also exacerbate an existing health problem.

The idea that stress is all bad, however, is a misunderstanding. Unlike sheep, we humans need a high amount of stimulation to motivate and keep us going. It sharpens our senses and helps us to adapt to our environment. Indeed, without the 'spice of life' we begin to feel down-hearted. So, whether we are suffering from the strain of living in the fast track, or the burden of a monotonous existence, in either situation we feel we have no control over our life so we experience distress. The secret of maintaining well-being is to find just the right level of stimulation and relaxation to make life interesting and fulfilling, and this balance is different for every individual.

The Role of Aromatherapy

Aromatherapy is one of the finest treatments available for reducing stress and uplifting mood. Ideally, combine home treatments with the occasional professional aromatherapy massage.

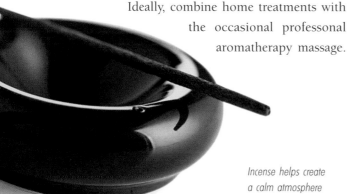

Incense helps create a calm atmosphere

PLEASING AROMAS

When using aromatherapy for mind and spirit, aroma preference is even more important than usual. The recipes given in this chapter work beautifully if the aromas are perceived as pleasing. If, however, you dislike a particular blend, the treatment is unlikely to be effective. Always be prepared to experiment with combinations of appropriate oils (refer to the Quick Guide to Essential Oils, page 134) until you find the blend which you like most. Of course, a single essential oil can be effective if it feels right for your needs.

The beauty of aromatherapy is that it combines the medicinal properties of nature's essential oils with the soul-caressing properties of scent. The mere act of blending mood-enhancing aromas awakens our creative instincts. Add gentle music and pleasing surroundings, and we also heighten our sense of hearing and sight. Apply with tender loving care, and we are nurtured on every level of our being.

The following aromatherapy treatments are for a number of common stress-related ailments. As an adjunct to the treatments suggested for each condition, it is helpful to take other steps to promote relaxation and revitalization. The most effective techniques include yoga, t'ai chi, free-expressive dance and various forms of meditation. For some people, a relaxation tape is the most effective and accessible option.

Anxiety and Stress

Although the term 'stress' may be applied in a general sense to indicate almost any state of distress or anxiety, it is commonly associated with the 'fight or flight' hormones – adrenaline and nor-adrenaline. These chemicals prepare us to resist ('fight') or avoid ('flight') attack. In modern life, it is not always possible to deal with stress in this way, so we bottle up our true feelings. As a result, there is no direct outlet for the effects of adrenaline. The longer the 'stressed out' feeling remains, the more potentially harmful it can be, eventually compromising physical and emotional well-being.

Foods rich in B vitamins benefit the nervous system, so include bananas, nuts, green vegetables and whole grains in your diet. Oats are nourishing to a frantic nervous system too. During particularly stressful periods, it can be beneficial to take a good vitamin B-complex supplement (dosage as directed on the label). Drastically reduce your intake of caffeine and instead drink plenty of bottled water and soothing herb teas such as chamomile, vervain, lemon balm, orange flower and rose petal.

For some people, strenuous exercise is the most effective way to dissipate stress, for others, relaxation techniques work best. Often the best approach is to combine strenuous activity and stillness. Aromatherapy can be used as an enjoyable supportive measure.

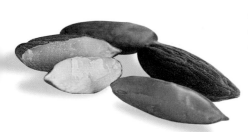

Nuts, including almonds, are a good source of vitamin B

Essential Oil Concentrates for Stress and Anxiety

The first blend contains deeply resonating notes to help curb the hyperactive kind of stress, often the initial phase before exhaustion sets in. The second blend has a lighter, energizing quality and may be more helpful for nervous exhaustion.

◉ Tranquil Sea

20 drops mandarin essential oil
8 drops neroli (or petitgrain) essential oil
1 drop spikenard (or vetiver) essential oil
2 drops frankincense essential oil
8 drops clary sage essential oil
6 drops lavender essential oil

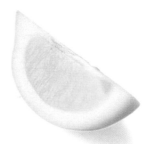

Lemon oil acts as an energizer

Put the essential oils in a dark glass bottle and shake well.

◉ Vibrant Sky

15 drops bergamot essential oil
8 drops lemon essential oil
6 drops rosemary essential oil
6 drops petitgrain essential oil
4 drops rose otto (or geranium) essential oil
6 drops Virginian cedarwood essential oil

Put the essential oils into a small dark glass bottle and shake well.

The essential oil concentrates are measured by the drop and used in the following recipes and applications.

Land of Milk and Honey Bath

For this bath, the milk and honey moisturizes and nourishes stressed skin. You may also wish to burn candles and play soothing or energizing music (depending on your need) to enhance your enjoyment.

300ml goat's milk
1 tablespoon liquid honey
6 drops of essential oil concentrate.

Add the milk and honey while the water is still running. Once the bath has been filled, add the essential oil and swish around to disperse.

Massage Oil

25ml sweet almond oil
8–10 drops essential oil concentrate

Funnel the sweet almond oil into a dark glass bottle, add the essential oil and shake well. Apply after your bath or shower. Although the oil may be massaged into the whole of your body, you may prefer to concentrate on the area which is especially sensitive to psychic distress: the solar plexus region (the area of the body where the ribs make a 'V' shape), the abdomen and the soles of the feet.

Vaporizer Blends

Here are some delightfully relaxing and uplifting blends. Alternatively, you may prefer to add a couple of drops of 'Tranquil Sea' or 'Vibrant Sky' concentrate to the water-filled dish of the vaporizer.

Sunset

Rosewater
1 drop ylang-ylang essential oil
1 drop lime essential oil

Fill the vaporizer dish with rosewater, then add the essential oils.

Sunrise

Orange flower water
1 drop lemon essential oil
1 drop orange essential oil
1 drop grapefruit essential oil
2 drops Virginian cedarwood

Fill the vaporizer dish with orangeflower water, then add the essential oils.

Dry Inhalation

For this method, you may wish to use one of the essential oil concentrates given above. Otherwise, choose your favourite relaxing oil from the list in the Quick Guide to Essential Oils (page 134). Put a few drops of essential oil onto a tissue and inhale at intervals as required.

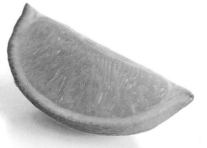

lime combines with ylang-ylang and rosewater for the Sunset blend

Depression

Depression is a normal response to crisis, emotional upheaval or excessive stress. But long-term depression with no obvious cause usually indicates an underlying physical or psychiatric illness, and needs professional help. Post-natal depression should also be regarded as serious if it lingers for more than a month or two after childbirth. Your doctor may be able to put you in touch with a counsellor or psychotherapist.

It is also worth consulting a nutritional therapist. In many cases of depression, food allergies or intolerances are the culprits, and once identified, the problem can be remedied. Milder depression, triggered by an unhappy situation in your life, can be successfully treated at home using dietary measures, herbal remedies and aromatherapy. The most important foods are complex carbohydrates such as wholegrain bread, oats, pasta, rice and potatoes which encourage the brain to produce the 'feel-good' hormone, serotonin. But avoid alcohol as this interrupts sleep and intensifies depression by lowering the brain's levels of serotonin.

Herb teas with uplifting properties include lemon balm, lavender and vervain. But the most important herbal remedy is hypericum or St John's wort, which has been shown to be more effective for mild to moderate depression than conventional antidepressant drugs. Hypericum tablets are available from pharmacies and health stores

Vitamin supplements can be used to support your diet

(take as directed). Regular and enjoyable exercise is important too – such as a walk in the park every day – as this triggers the release of endorphins and encephalins which elevate mood.

Essential Oil Concentrate for Depression

⬥ Woodland Ascent

2 drops cistus (or vetiver) essential oil
10 drops Canadian balsam essential oil
10 drops Virginian cedarwood essential oil
8 drops bergamot essential oil
6 drops lemon essential oil
8 drops clary sage essential oil

Put the essential oils into a small dark glass bottle and shake well. This aromatic formula may be measured by the drop and used for baths, massage, vaporization and dry inhalation (see recommended quantities given on page 14). Otherwise, enjoy the blends which follow.

⬥ Green Clay Bath

A green clay bath stimulates the circulation and lymph flow, making you feel tingly and alive. This bath may be taken once or twice a week. If taken more frequently, it can be drying to the skin. At other times, simply enjoy aromatic baths without the clay. Burn candles and play uplifting music to enhance the experience.

250g green clay
2 drops rosemary essential oil
2 drops lemon essential oil
2 drops coriander essential oil

Run a comfortably hot bath, then mix in the green clay. Add the essential oils and swish around to disperse.

● Massage Oil

25ml sweet almond oil
2 drops frankincense essential oil
2 drops neroli essential oil
5 drops bergamot

Funnel the sweet almond oil into a dark glass bottle, add the essential oil and shake well. Apply after your bath or shower. Although the oil may massaged into the whole of your body, you may prefer to concentrate on the area which is especially sensitive to the effects of emotional distress: the solar plexus region, the abdomen and the soles of the feet.

● Vaporizing Blend

Rosewater and orange flower water
1 drop rosemary essential oil
1 drop lemongrass essential oil

Fill the vaporizer dish with a 50:50 mix of rosewater and orange flower water, then add the essential oils.

● Dry Inhalation

For this method, you may wish to use the 'Woodland Ascent' concentrate given above. Otherwise, choose from the list given in the Quick Guide to Essential Oils.

Put a few drops of essential oil on a tissue and inhale at intervals as required.

Seasonal Affective Disorder

'Winter depression' affects many people to a greater or lesser degree. Shorter days and longer nights cause an imbalance in brain chemistry, principally a decrease in the 'feel good' hormone, serotonin, and an imbalance of the sleep hormone, melatonin. As a result, sufferers experience distressing symptoms such as fatigue, overeating, an increased desire to sleep (upwards of 10 hours a night), depression, anxiety, irritability, loss of libido and moodiness.

To encourage the production of stimulating catecholamine brain hormones, nutritional therapists recommend that sufferers eat more protein foods during winter, such as fish, chicken and soya products, along with plenty of vitamin-rich fresh fruits and vegetables. The most effective herbal remedy for all types of depression is St John's wort or hypericum which is available from pharmacies and health stores (take as directed).

If you suffer from a mild form of the winter blues and are forced to spend a great deal of time indoors, it is worth investing in some full-spectrum lighting, which mimics natural daylight as it contains all the colours of the rainbow. Severe cases respond best to very bright light emitted from a full-spectrum light box (these are small enough to be placed on a desk or worktop).

Try a friction rub to alleviate winter depression

Light therapy, which helps to maintain a balance between serotonin and melatonin production, has an impressive 85 per cent success rate. The boxes are obtainable from specialist mail order suppliers (ask at your local health store or natural therapy centre for a contact address).

Aromatherapy is an excellent supportive treatment for lifting mood. As well as the friction rub given below, the treatments suggested for depression (see page 97) and stress (see page 95) may also be helpful.

● Friction Rub for the Winter Blues

Try this sunny blend to lift your spirits and improve circulation. To increase its beneficial effects, use in combination with dry skin brushing (see page 20).

● Sol

20ml macerated hypericum oil
 (or extra virgin olive oil)
20ml sweet almond oil
2 drops palmarosa essential oil
2 drops lemongrass essential oil
4 drops coriander essential oil
8 drops rosemary essential oil

Funnel the hypericum and sweet almond oil into a dark glass bottle, add the essential oils and shake well. Apply after your daily shower, using brisk hand-over-hand strokes towards the heart to stimulate circulation and lymph flow.

Mental Fatigue

This condition is especially common in writers, office workers and students studying for their exams. Try to take regular breaks and provide for compensatory physical exercise, preferably in the fresh air. It also helps to do something 'grounding' or practical such as gardening, cooking or perhaps a blitz on the housework. Laughter is a wonderful antidote, so watch a funny film or play – or meet up with friends and have a good belly laugh! When you return to your mental work, try one of the following blends to promote clarity of thought.

● Einstein (for the vaporizer)

2 drops peppermint essential oil
2 drop rosemary essential oil
2 drops clary sage essential oil

Fill the vaporizer dish with water, then add the essential oils.

● Eureka! (dry inhalation)

1 drop myrtle (or eucalyptus) essential oil
1 drop lemon essential oil

Put the essential oils on a tissue and inhale at intervals as required.

Eucalyptus oil aids concentration

Palpitations

Palpitations are a fluttering in the chest, caused by a rapid or irregular heartbeat. Pounding of the heart other than after exercise, emotional shock or excitement needs further investigation. It may be the result of food allergy, hormonal fluctuation, chronic high blood pressure, or consuming nicotine or caffeine. It may also indicate a heart problem. Provided the problem is stress-related, then aromatherapy and herbal remedies can certainly help. It is advisable to have a medical check-up first.

Essential Oil Concentrate for Palpitations

Still Waters

10 drops rose otto essential oil
5 drops frankincense
10 drops mandarin essential oil
10 drops petitgrain essential oil

Put the essential oils into a small dark glass bottle and shake well. This aromatic formula may be measured by the drop and used for baths, massage, vaporization and dry inhalation as suggested below.

Aromatic Bath (as a preventative treatment)

Add six drops of the 'Still Waters' concentrate to the bath after it has been filled, then swish around to disperse.

Massage Oil (as a preventative treatment)

25ml sweet almond oil
8–10 drops 'Still Waters' concentrate

Put the sweet almond oil into a dark glass bottle, then add the essential oils and shake well. Apply after a bath or shower, concentrating on the areas which are especially sensitive to the effects of emotional distress: the solar plexus region, the abdomen and the soles of the feet.

Vaporizer Blend (as a preventative treatment)

Relax in the evenings with this room fragrance. Alternatively, add the same quantity of 'Still Waters' concentrate to the orange flower water.

Orange flower water
2 drops frankincense essential oil
2 drops lavender essential oil

Fill the vaporizer dish with orange flower water, then add the essential oil.

Dry Inhalation (to quell an attack)

This method is for when you are experiencing palpitations. Any of the oils recommended for palpitations may be used (see the Quick Guide to Essential Oils) or use the 'Still Waters' concentrate. Put one or two drops of essential oil on a tissue, then inhale the aroma slowly and deeply.

Migraine

A migraine is a very distressing and debilitating heachache accompanied by altered vision, nausea and sometimes vomiting. There are many possible causes, which usually include stress and severe tension in the neck and shoulders. The commonest food triggers are cheese, chocolate, coffee, strong tea, red wine and yeast products. Personality and character may also be a direct link; migraine sufferers tend to be anxious and hard-working, perhaps also perfectionists.

Although home treatments can help ease symptoms, professional help from a nutritional therapist is strongly advised. As a preventative, ask a friend or partner to give you a regular aromatherapy massage, especially to the head, neck and shoulders. Ideally, also have a weekly or fortnightly professional full-body massage to reduce stress levels. During an attack, most people benefit from lying down in a darkened room until symptoms ease. The best herbal remedy is feverfew, which is most effective as a preventative. Feverfew tablets are available from pharmacies and health food stores (take as directed). Alternatively try the tea recipes suggested below.

◗ Aromatic Compress for Migraine

Some people benefit from an icy application, others experience relief from a warm compress. So you will need to experiment to find which application brings the most relief.

600ml (1pt) icy cold or tolerably warm water
3 drops lavender essential oil
1 drop sweet marjoram essential oil

Pour the water into a bowl, then add the essential oils and swish around to disperse. Soak two pieces of folded cotton fabric in the water, wring it out, and apply to the forehead and back of the neck. Leave in place until the compress reaches body temperature, then reapply if necessary.

◗ Herb Teas for Migraine

(using dried herbs)
2 teaspoons dried thyme
1 teaspoon dried sage
2 teaspoons dried peppermint
1 ltr (2pts) boiling water

Put the herbs into a china teapot, add the boiling water and allow to steep for 15 minutes. Take a teacupful every two hours until you experience relief.

(using fresh herbs)
10g fresh lemon balm
10g fresh basil
10g fresh rosemary
600ml (1pt) boiling water

Preparation and dosage as above.

Chocolate can trigger a migraine

Tension headache

Although not as severe as a full-blown migraine, tension headaches can be incapacitating. The first step is to find ways to reduce stress in your life, a relaxation tape may be the most accessible method. As with all stress-related problems, regular aromatherapy massage is a marvellous preventative treatment. Ask a friend or partner to massage your head, neck and shoulders. Ideally, also have a fortnightly or monthly professional full-body massage. To treat a tension headache, try the herbal blends suggested below. You may also find the following aromatherapy treatments helpful.

◉ Cold Compress

600ml cold water
1 drop peppermint essential oil
2 drops lavender essential oil

Pour the water into a bowl, then add the essential oils and swish around to disperse. Soak a piece of folded cotton fabric in the water, wring it out, apply to the forehead and lie down for 15 minutes.

◉ Massage Oil
This blend contains a high concentration of essential oil for local application. If you have sensitive skin, use the dry inhalation method instead.

1 teaspoon sweet almond oil
3 drops peppermint essential oil
3 drops lavender essential oil

Mix the oils together in an eggcup, then massage into the temples and around the back of the neck.

◉ Dry Inhalation
Put a few drops of essential oil on a tissue and inhale every few minutes until you experience relief. The most effective oil for this method is peppermint. However, if you dislike peppermint try lavender, or any other essential oil recommended for headache (refer to the Quick Guide to Essential Oils on page 134).

◉ Herb Teas for Tension Headache

(using dried herbs)
1 teaspoon dried linden blossom
1 teaspoon dried chamomile flowers
1 teaspoon dried lavender flowers
500ml (1pt) boiling water

Put the herbs into a china teapot, add the boiling water and allow to steep for 15 minutes. Take a teacupful every two hours until you experience relief.

(using fresh herbs)
10g fresh peppermint or spearmint
10g fresh basil
10g fresh lavender

Prepare as per Dried Herbal Tea.

Peppermint to relieve tension headache

Insomnia

There are a number of aromatic herbs and essential oils which will help sufferers of insomnia. Of the herbs, the most valuable are hops, lavender, valerian and passiflora. These are often included in proprietary herbal compound tablets which are available from health stores and pharmacies (take as dir-ected) or try the soporific tea listed below. The most valuable essential oil is lavender, whose soporific properties have been validated through clinical studies. A single drop of undiluted lavender oil may be put on each corner of your pillow (the undiluted oil will not leave a permenant stain on cotton fabric). The following aromatic treatments may also be helpful.

Essential Oil Concentrate for Insomnia

◦ Dream Time

20 drops lavender essential oil
8 drops Roman chamomile
  (or 6 drops rose otto) essential oil
10 drops clary sage essential oil

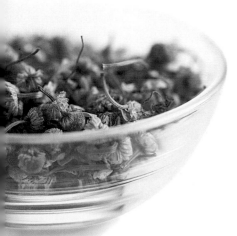

Add chamomile to a blend for insomnia

Put the essential oils into a small dark glass bottle and shake well. Measure by the drop for use in the f ollowing treatments.

◦ Evening Aromatic Bath

Add six drops of the 'Dream Time' concentrate to a comfortably warm (not hot) bath shortly before bedtime. Burn candles and play soft music to enhance the effect.

◦ Massage Oil

25ml sweet almond oil
8 drops 'Dream Time' concentrate

Funnel the sweet almond oil into a dark glass bottle, add the essential oil and shake well. Apply after your evening bath. Massage into the solar plexus region (just below the ribs). Better still, have someone give you a soothing back massage about an hour before going to bed.

◦ Soporific Herb Tea (helps promote restful sleep)

1 teaspoon dried chamomile flowers
1 teaspoon dried orange flowers
1 teaspoon linden blossom
600ml (1pt) boiled water

Put the herbs into a china teapot, add the boiling water and allow to steep for 15 minutes. Take a teacupful three times a day.

EMOTIONAL HEALING WITH ESSENTIAL OILS

There are several different schools of thought regarding the emotional effects of essential oils. Some practitioners believe that a given oil will always engender a predictable effect upon the emotions; while others (like myself) believe that the emotional effects are largely idiosyncratic – albeit that we can make a few generalizations.

At risk of adding to the mystery surrounding the psycho-spiritual aspects of aromatherapy, in my own experience people are usually drawn to the essential oils which reflect their mood or personality. When experiencing acute emotional distress such as anger or nervousness, for example, most people are comforted by a light-bodied oil such as lemon or lavender, rather than a heavy and tenacious aroma like patchouli. On the other hand, when suffering from prolonged psychic distress resulting in feelings of despondency and despair, less volatile 'grounding' oils like cedarwood, Canadian balsam, juniper berry or pine are often chosen.

With regard to personality types, extroverts (when feeling in good form) tend to be attracted to light-hearted aromas with little tenacity, while more introverted people (when not acutely distressed) usually prefer rich, lingering aromas.

So the oil (or blend) that best matches the energetic nature of your mood or personality is more likely to gain access to your innermost being – and in so doing, dissipate psychic distress. Exactly how an aromatherapy blend can possibly achieve such an alchemical feat is open to conjecture, though it does compare with the homoeopathic Law of Similars, that 'like cures like'. But rather than launching into an esoteric explanation, it is far better to explore this fascinating aspect of aromatherapy for yourself.

◆ Delving Deeper into Aroma

Since none of the senses is so easily fatigued as the sense of smell, you will need to limit you smelling explorations to about four oils in one sitting, certainly no more than six. It can also be helpful to record in a notebook your feelings, recollections and associated imagery.

When exploring aromas to discover their generalized effects on your psyche, choose a time when you are feeling calm and receptive. Sit in a comfortable position in a quiet, well-ventilated room which is free of any cooking smells or other intrusive odours. Mix a few drops of your chosen essential oil with half a teaspoon of sweet almond oil. Dip one end of a smelling paper (available from essential oil suppliers) or a thin strip of blotting paper into the aromatic mixture. It is also a good idea to write the name of the oil on the dry end of the paper, especially when exploring more than two oils. Waft the smelling strip around to encourage vaporization, then inhale the fragrance

Enjoy the whole process of aromatherapy – from buying equipment to applying the oils

slowly and deeply, allowing your-self to experience its effect fully.

Stay with the fragrance for a couple of minutes. What does the aroma make you think of? Is it a feeling, memory or image you would like to have more often? Write down your impressions, even if this amounts to single words like 'clean', 'cheery', 'airy', 'apples', 'woody', 'medicinal', or even in terms of sounds, tastes, textures, colours and shapes. You might even feel inspired to paint or draw whatever imagery the aroma may evoke.

At other times, when you are experiencing some form of emotional disharmony, explore these aromas once more (or perhaps a few different oils as well). Again, write down your impressions of each oil. If you have already explored the same oil while feeling in good spirits, make a note of any changes you may be experiencing now. If you are a woman you will find it especially interesting to record your responses at different phases of the menstrual cycle.

◗ Moon Shadow Aromas

Having emphasized the importance of working with aromas you enjoy, there is one exception to the rule. Should an aroma make you feel uncom-fortable in any way, perhaps evoking an unhappy memory or a disturbing image, even this can be used as a healing tool.

Begin by giving yourself permission to respond to the aroma therapeutically. This is achieved simply by telling yourself it will be a healing

Create the right mood for applying essential oils

experience. Of course, don't attempt to work with an oil if it makes you feel nauseous. Such extreme reactions aside, provided the oil is perceived as tolerable, it may be useful for emotional healing.

On inhaling the aroma, try to write about your feelings in as much detail as possible. Simply allow one impression to lead into another and continue writing until you come to a natural end. If you relax into this exercise you will be surprised how easily the words flow on to the page. Even though the prose may seem disjointed, it is by viewing a dark or disturbing feeling in the light of conscious awareness that it becomes less threatening, perhaps totally disem-powered. For example, have you ever written a venomous letter to someone, but decided in the end not to send it? You probably felt a great deal better for having vented your wrath, and relieved that there were no embarrassing repercussions!

◗ Healing Emotional Disharmony

On pages 106 to 107 you will see a reference chart for healing emotional disharmony. This chart represents the possibilites for emotional healing and is based on the the law of averages. Your own responses may be quite different, so always be guided by your sense of smell and allow it take you where it will. Your chosen oils may be used in the bath, in a massage blend, a vaporizer or inhaled from a tissue (as recommended for depression, insomnia and other stress-related conditions discussed earlier in this chapter).

HEALING EMOTIONAL DISHARMONY

EMOTIONAL STATE	SUGGESTED HEALING AROMAS
Grief	Rose, marjoram, frankincense, pine, cypress, Canadian balsam, sandalwood, spikenard, helichrysum, vetiver.
Shock	Sudden emotional trauma: Lavender, lemon, bergamot, clary sage, neroli, peppermint, petitgrain, rosemary, eucalyptus, myrtle, rose. Lingering effects of past emotional trauma: Frankincense, sandalwood, spikenard, cistus, Canadian balsam, cedarwood (Atlas or Virginian), pine, juniper berry, rose.
Anger, irritability and frustration	Acute distress: Bergamot (and other citrus oils), clary sage, peppermint, lavender, mandarin, pine, Roman chamomile, geranium, petitgrain. Deep-rooted anger and frustration: Rose, cedarwood (Atlas or Virginian), Canadian balsam, cypress, frankincense, ylang-ylang, helichrysum, marjoram, neroli, spikenard, sandalwood.
Mood swings	Bergamot, mandarin, Roman chamomile, frankincense, geranium, juniper berry, lavender, lemon, rose, sandalwood, ylang-ylang.
Despondency, despair, pessimism	Initial stages of healing process: Lavender, spikenard, sandalwood, Canadian balsam, cedarwood (Atlas or Virginian), cistus, clary sage, frankincense, cypress.

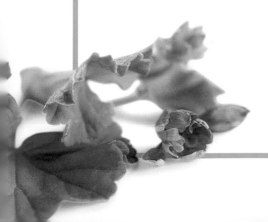

EMOTIONAL STATE	SUGGESTED HEALING AROMAS
Despondency, despair, pessimism	Later stages of healing process: Bergamot (and other citrus oils), coriander, geranium, neroli, lemongrass, rose, rosemary, ylang-ylang.
Worry, nervous tension, restlessness	Bergamot (and other citrus oils), Roman chamomile, Canadian balsam, cedarwood (Atlas or Virginian), cypress, frankincense, lavender, neroli, petitgrain, clary sage, myrtle, sandalwood, geranium, rose.
Poor concentration	Peppermint, lavender, myrtle, cardamom, coriander, cypress, eucalyptus, frankincense, lemon, lime, lemongrass, pine, rosemary.
Confusion and indecision	Bergamot (and other citrus oils), cypress, eucalyptus, frankincense, geranium, myrtle, pine, peppermint, rosemary.
Fearfulness	Frankincense, cypress, cedarwood (Atlas or Virginian), Canadian balsam, juniper berry, marjoram, rose, sandalwood, vetiver, palmarosa, lemongrass, spikenard, lavender.
Emotionally induced loss of libido	Rose, ylang-ylang, ginger, coriander, clary sage, sandalwood, patchouli, cardamom, neroli, black pepper, juniper berry, Atlas cedarwood.

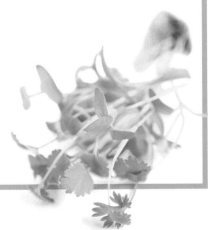

Meditation and the Spirit

Meditation is a state of relaxed alertness, of being fully present in the moment. Its ultimate aim is to facilitate communcation with the spiritual aspect of our being – the all-wise aspect that manifests itself in those rare moments of inspiration and clarity when we experience profound insight into the meaning and purpose of our existence. The best way to learn meditation is from an experienced teacher, although there are also many excellent books on the subject. The blends given below may be used to enhance meditation. If you are a newcomer to spiritual contemplation, this section includes a simple meditation on the rhythm of the breath and other suggestions for nurturing the soul.

MEDITATION BLENDS FOR THE VAPORIZER

For meditational purposes, by far the most pleasing form of vaporizer is the simple ceramic candle-heated variety. The elements of earth (the ceramic pot itself), air (the aromatic vapour), fire (the candle flame) and water combine to create a naturally peaceful ambience. For all the recipes given below, simply add the essential oils to the water-filled dish of the vaporizer, then light the candle.

◊ Moonlight on the Lake

1 drop cistus essential oil
2 drops petitgrain essential oil
1 drop cypress
2 drops clary sage essential oil
1 drops frankincense essential oil

◊ Jewel in the Lotus

1 drop spikenard essential oil
2 drops Scots pine essential oil
2 drops lavender essential oil
1 drop lemon essential oil
1 drop lime essential oil

◊ Tranquillity

1 drop vetiver essential oil
2 drops petitgrain essential oil
2 drops clary sage essential oil
2 drops Canadian balsam
 (or Virginian cedarwood) essential oil

◊ Wind through Reeds

2 drops frankincense essential oil
2 drops bergamot essential oil
1 drop lemon essential oil
2 drops Scots pine essential oil

◊ Temple Bells

1 drop peppermint
2 drops clary sage
2 drops Virginian
 cedarwood
2 drops sandalwood

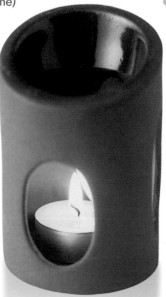

Use vaporizer blends to aid meditation

CONTEMPLATING THE BEAUTY OF A FLOWER

Here is a simple nature attunement exercise that you may enjoy during your precious moments of solitude.

Go out into the garden and pick a selection of flowers, including some fragrant blooms. If you don't have a garden, treat yourself to a bunch of seasonal flowers from a florist. Begin by breathing in the fragrance, focusing your attention on the delightful sensation. Now run your fingertips over the cool, silken petals. Next look at the blooms through a magnifying glass in sunlight. You will be enraptured by the translucent beauty revealed in close-up: delicately-veined petals, mysterious crevices glistening with moisture, hues within hues, the perfection of form, the sheer vitality of the blooms. From this perspective familiar garden flowers suddenly take on a whole new meaning – transporting the senses to other dimensions.

CREATE A SEASONAL ALTAR IN YOUR HOME

A beautiful way to remind yourself of the special-ness of life and nature is to create an 'altar' or sacred space in your home. An altar is a spiritual focal point, an aid to stilling the mind and refresh-ing the soul. This sacred space may be created on a window sill, a small table in front of a mirror, a mantlepiece or the top of a wooden chest. Trust your intuition and find the space that resonates with your inner being. Decorate the space with such things as pebbles, crystals, driftwood and seasonal flowers. To this arrangement, add an appealing essential oil burner, and float rose petals and floating candles in an attractive water-filled bowl. During autumn and winter, you might like to float autumn leaves, tiny larch cones, berries and sprigs of evergreen. Just light the candles in the evening for an enchanting effect.

Meditation on the Breath

This ancient breathing meditation engenders clarity of thought and inner peace. Find a quiet place where you will not be disturbed for at least 15 minutes. Sit in a comfortable but upright position with your feet flat on the floor, hands resting in your lap. Or sit crossed-legged on the floor if you are accustomed to this position. Wear loose, comfortable clothing so as not to restrict your breathing.

Close your eyes and become aware of your breathing. Make no effort to control the breath, simply focus on its ebb and flow, paying special attention to the stillpoint before each inhalation. And now on every out-breath, count 'one' and then 'two' and so on up to 10. Remember to count only on the out-breath. Once you reach 10, go back to the beginning. If you lose count or your mind wanders (as it surely will), do not become irritated but simply start count-ing again with one. Continue to count for about 10 minutes or until you experience a sense of tranquillity.

Flowers and candles have a calming effect on the mind

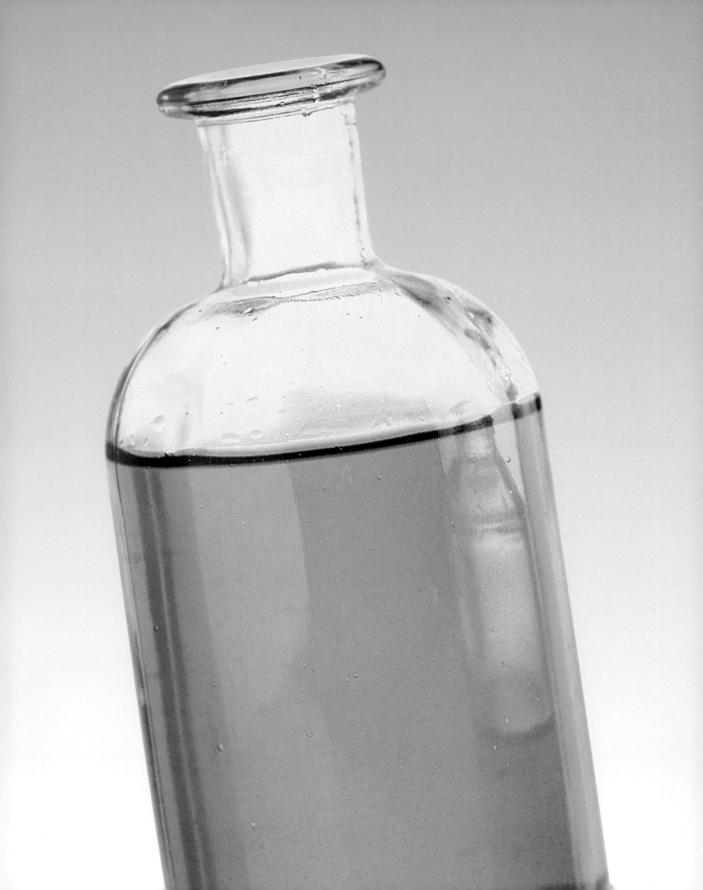

Directory of Essential Oils

When we are dealing with an essential oil and its odoriferance, we are dealing directly with a vital force and entering the very heart of the alchemy of creation.

MARGUERITE MAURY

The Secret of Life and Youth (Macdonald & Co., 1964)

The essential oils profiled in the directory are arranged in alphabetical order according to their Latin or botanical names. This is because the common names of plants differ from one region to another whereas the botanical names are recognized throughout the world.

Even though the exact botanical source may be of little interest to the home user, for professional purposes it serves as a guide to the probable chemical composition of the chosen oil, and thus the oil's therapeutic properties. For instance, although there are several types of pine oil available to aromatherapists, only that which is extracted from *Pinus sylvestris* (Scots pine) is safe for home use – that is to say, provided the usual safety precautions when dealing with the oil are taken into account.

Each profile begins with a brief description of the plant and its habitat, which is especially interesting for those readers who are unfamiliar with exotic essential oil-yielding plants such as frankincense from North Africa, patchouli from Indonesia, ylang-ylang from Madagasgar and spikenard from India. Indeed, aromatic plants are found all over the world and essential oil production is an international industry.

Information on each essence also includes the method of extraction; characteristic colour and viscosity of the oil; odour description and common emotional effects; aromatherapy uses and aesthetic blending. Any precautions to be observed in relation to the use of a particular essential oil are given in the caution note at the end of the relevant aromatic profile.

Abies balsamea

Canadian Balsam

Family: Pinaceae

A tall, graceful evergreen tree native to North America. It forms blisters of oleo resin (the so-called balsam) on the trunk and branches. The essential oil is captured by steam distillation of the hardened oleo resin. The oil is usually only available from specialist suppliers, but worth seeking out. It is a virtually colourless liquid with a sweet, soft-balsamic, pine-like aroma. The odour effect is warming, comforting and energizing.

Aromatherapy Uses
Burns, cuts, wounds, bronchitis, catarrh, coughs, sore throat, mild depression, anxiety, nervous tension and other stress-related states. Ideal as a vaporizing oil for respiratory ailments or, alternatively, for mood-enhancement.

Blending Guide
Middle note; medium odour intensity.
Blends well with pine, cedarwood, frankincense, sandalwood, juniper berry, cypress, lemon, clary sage.

Boswellia carteri

Frankincense/Olibanum

Family: Burseraceae

The oil is extracted by steam distillation of frankincense 'tears' – little pieces of solidified oleo gum resin – which exude from natural fissures in the bark of the small tree. Frankincense is native to the arid regions of Arabia and North Africa. The essential oil is colourless to pale yellow with a warm, balsamic, camphoric aroma. Unlike most other essential oils, the aroma of frankincense improves with age. Its odour effect is warming, head-clearing and calming. Commonly used in a vaporizer as a meditation aid.

Aromatherapy Uses
Skin care (particularly mature skin), acne, abscesses, scars, wounds, haemorrhoids, respiratory ailments such as asthma, bronchitis, coughs, catarrh, laryngitis, cystitis, arthritic and rheumatic pain, painful menstruation, spotting between periods, PMS, nervous tension and other stress-related states.

Blending Guide
Base note; high odour intensity.
Blends well with citrus oils, coriander and other spice oils, Canadian balsam, cedarwood, cypress, geranium, juniper berry, lavender, neroli, palmarosa, patchouli, petitgrain, rose, spikenard, sandalwood, vetiver.

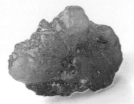

CAUTION
Highly odoriferous, so use in the lowest recommended concentrations.

Calendula officinalis

Calendula/Marigold

Family: *Asteraceae (Compositae)*

NB: The product described here is not an essential oil, but an infused or macerated oil. Available from aromatherapy and herbal suppliers.

An attractive herb with bright orange or yellow daisy-like flowers. Native to Mediterranean countries, but cultivated worldwide. The plant produces too little essential oil to make distillation commercially viable. Instead, the flowerheads are macerated in a vegetable oil base (usually sunflower or olive). It is golden yellow with a dry, honey-like aroma.

● Aromatherapy Uses
Use undiluted for sore, inflamed and itchy skin conditions, including eczema, nappy rash, athlete's foot, sore and cracked nipples in nursing mothers, minor burns and bruises. Helps prevent stretch marks during pregnancy. Good for dry, sensitive skin prone to thead veins. May also reduce inflammation in varicose veins.

● Blending Guide
The aroma and anti-inflammatory properties can be enhanced with the addition of any of the following oils: chamomile (Roman or German), helichrysum, lavender, rose otto. Usual ratio is one drop of essential oil per 20–30ml calendula infusion.

● CAUTION
Not to be confused with essential oil of Tagete (*Tagetes minuta*), the Mexican marigold, which is potentially toxic.

Cananga odorata var. *genuina*

Ylang-ylang

Family: *Annonaceae*

Ylang-ylang (pronounced ee-lang ee-lang) is a tropical tree with large glossy leaves and intensely fragrant yellow blooms. Most of the oil is produced in Madagascar, Réunion and the Comoros Islands and it is captured by steam distillation of the fresh flowers. There are several grades: ylang-ylang extra, and ylang-ylang one, two and three. There is also a 'complete' oil. Most aromatherapists favour 'extra' and 'complete' grades because of their superior fragrances.

Ylang-ylang 'complete' represents the total or 'unfractionated' oil which is collected at the end of a long process of distillation. All grades of oil are pale yellow or virtually colourless. The extra and complete grades have a fragrance reminiscent of almonds and jasmine combined, while the other fractions are harsh and woody by comparison. The odour effect of a good quality ylang-ylang is warming and intoxicating, and reputedly aphrodisiac.

● Aromatherapy Uses
High blood pressure, palpitations, mild depression, insomnia, PMS, other stress-related states.

● Blending Guide
Middle to base note; high odour intensity.
Used sparingly, ylang ylang blends well with other florals, black pepper and other spices, citrus oils, frankincense, geranium, sandalwood, vetiver.

● CAUTION
Highly odoriferous, so use in the lowest recommended concentrations.

Cedrus atlantica

Cedarwood

Family: *Pinaceae*

A hardy evergreen conifer producing an abundance of cylindrical cones. The tree is native to the Atlas Mountains of Algeria and Morocco, but extensively cultivated in Europe and North America. Most of the oil is produced in Morocco and is captured by steam distillation of the wood, stumps and sawdust. It is a dark amber, viscous liquid with a tenaceous, sweet, woody aroma. Its odour effect is warming, calming and reputedly aphrodisiac.

◖ Aromatherapy Uses
Acne, oily skin and hair, dandruff, fungal infections, arthritis and rheumatism, coughs, bronchitis, catarrh, emotional symptoms of PMS, nervous tension and other stress-related states. May also be used to repel moths.

◖ Blending Guide
Base note; medium odour intensity.
Blends well with bergamot and other citrus oils, geranium, lemongrass, palmarosa, cistus, clary sage, cypress, frankincense, juniper berry, pine, coriander, Canadian balsam, neroli, rose, rosemary, vetiver, ylang-ylang.

◖ CAUTION
Avoid this during pregnancy. Ceadrwood oil may irritate sensitive skin, so use it in the lowest recommended concentrations.

Chamaemelum nobile

Chamomile, Roman

Family: *Asteraceae (Compositae)*

This small, stocky herb with feathery leaves and daisy-like white flowers, is native to Europe and North America. The oil is extracted by steam distillation of the flower heads. It is pale yellow with a sweet aroma reminiscent of ripe apples. The odour effect is warming and calming.

◖ Aromatherapy Uses
Skin care (most skin-types), acne, inflamed skin conditions, earache, wounds, menstrual pain, PMS, headache, insomnia, nervous tension and other stress-related states.

◖ Blending Guide
Middle note; high odour intensity.
Blends well with citrus essences, carrot seed, clary sage, helichrysum, lavender, geranium, neroli, rose, ylang-ylang.

◖ CAUTION
Avoid skin applications during the first trimester of pregnancy as the oil reputedly stimulates menstruation. A highly odoriferous oil, so use in low concentrations of around one per cent. Due to the high price of Roman chamomile, there is a tendency for some essential oil suppliers to promote Moroccan chamomile (*Ormensis multicaulis*) as a cheaper alternative. Although the plant is distantly related to Roman chamomile and has a similar aroma, its medicinal properties have not been thoroughly investigated.

Cistus ladaniferus

Cistus

Family: *Cistaceae*

A small, sticky shrub with lance-shaped leaves and fragrant white flowers. The plant is native to the Mediterranean and the Middle East, and most of the oil is produced in Spain. It is captured by steam distillation of the crude gum (obtained by boiling the leaves and twigs in water), and sometimes the oil is extracted by distillation of the leaves and twigs directly. It is light amber with a penetrating and complex aroma, best described as sweet, dry-herbaceous with musky undertones. Its odour effect is warming, stimulating and uplifting; a reputed aphrodisiac.

◗ Aromatherapy Uses
Skin care (especially mature), bedsores, infected wounds, skin ulcers, bronchitis, coughs, colds and flu, as a fumigant when infectious illness is around, delayed periods outside pregnancy, as a meditation aid.

◗ Blending Guide
Middle to base note; extremely high odour intensity. Used sparingly, it blends well with cedarwood, coriander, clary sage, cypress, lavender, frankincense, juniper, pine, rose, lemon and other citrus oils, neroli, petitgrain, sandalwood, patchouli, vetiver.

◗ CAUTION
Avoid skin applications during pregnancy as it reputedly stimulates menstruation. Highly odoriferous; use in the lowest recommended concentrations.

Citrus aurantifolia

Lime

Family: *Rutaceae*

There are two methods of extraction: cold expression of the fresh peel, and steam distillation of the whole fruit. Although the expressed oil has a superior aroma, the distilled essence is the only type that can be used on the skin (see Caution). The distilled oil is virtually colourless, whereas the expressed essence is olive green. The scent is fresh, green and bitter. Its odour effect is uplifting and refreshing.

◗ Aromatherapy Uses
Colds and flu, poor circulation, high blood pressure, mild depression, nervous exhaustion and other stress-related states.

◗ Blending Guide
Top note; high odour intensity.
Lime oil blends well with other citrus essences, neroli, geranium, ginger and other spices, petitgrain, lavender, rosemary, clary sage, ylang-ylang.

◗ CAUTION
The expressed oil (but not the steam-distilled whole fruit oil) is highly phototoxic and must never be applied to skin, though it can be safely used in a vaporizer for mood-enhancement. The expressed oil has a short shelf-life and must be used within six months of opening. Distilled lime oil, however, will keep for at least 12 months after opening.
Use in the lowest recommended concentrations.

Citrus aurantium var. amara

Petitgrain

Family: Rutaceae

Other species: The essence is also extracted from *C.arrantium, subsp. aurantium.*

Petitgrain oil is captured by steam distillation of the leaves and twigs of the same tree that produces neroli oil. Most of the oil is produced in France, North Africa and Paraguay from semi-wild trees. It is pale yellow with a fresh, woody-herbaceous aroma reminiscent of neroli, but much less refined. The odour has a cooling and uplifting effect.

Aromatherapy Uses
Skin and hair care (oily), indigestion, insomnia, PMS, nervous exhaustion and other stress-related states.

Blending Guide
Top to middle note; moderately high odour intensity. Blends well with bergamot and other citrus oils, cedarwood, clary sage, clove, coriander, cypress, frankincense, geranium, lavender, neroli, palmarosa, spikenard, rose, rosemary, vetiver.

Citrus aurantium var. amara

Neroli

Family: *Rutaceae*

Other species: The essence is also extracted from *C. aurantium var. dulcis* or *C. aurantium subsp. aurantium.*

Neroli oil is captured by steam distillation of the freshly picked blossom of the bitter orange tree. Most of the oil is produced in Italy, Tunisia, France, Morocco and Egypt. Orange flower water – known as neroli hydrolat or hydrosol in the trade – is produced as a by-product of the distillation process. The essential oil is pale yellow, becoming darker with age, with a sweet-floral fragrance. Its odour effect is uplifting and soothing; a reputed aphrodisiac.

Aromatherapy Uses
Skin care (all skin types), as a preventative of stretch marks, palpitations, poor circulation, nervous diarrhoea, PMS, mild depression, nervous tension and other stress-related states. In aromatherapy, orange flower water is used mainly for skin care (for example, as a gentle toner).

Blending Guide
Middle note; moderately high odour intensity. Blends well with many oils, especially cedarwood, citrus essences, chamomile (Roman), clary sage, coriander, frankincense, geranium, lavender, petitgrain, rose, rosemary, spikenard, ylang-ylang.

Citrus bergamia

Bergamot

Family: *Rutaceae*

Bergamots are the small, greenish-yellow, orange-like fruits of a small citrus tree cultivated extensively in Italy and Sicily. The essential oil is extracted by cold expression of the fresh peel of the fruit. It is pale green with an aroma reminiscent of orange and grapefruit combined. Distilled bergamot FCF (see Caution), is virtually colourless with a less fruity aroma. The odour effect of bergamot is uplifting and refreshing.

Aromatherapy Uses
Colds and flu, cystitis, fever, emotional symptoms of PMS, sore throat, loss of appetite after illness, insect repellent, anxiety, mild depression and other stress-related states of mind.

Blending Guide
Top note; very low odour intensity.
Blends well with other citrus essences, cedarwood, chamomile (German and Roman), clary sage, coriander, lavender, neroli, cypress, frankincense, geranium, ginger, juniper, lemongrass, palmarosa, petitgrain, rose, rosemary, sandalwood, vetiver

CAUTION
The expressed oil is phototoxic. It should never be applied to skin shortly before exposure to natural or simulated sunlight as it can cause unsightly pigmentation and increase the risk of sunburn. Aromatherapists are increasingly using the rectified or distilled version known as bergamot FCF, which is non-phototoxic. Expressed bergamot oil is best used in a vaporizer for its mood-elevating effects.

Citrus limon

Lemon

Family: *Rutaceae*

A small evergreen tree producing fragrant white flowers, followed by the yellow fruit. Most of the oil is produced in Italy, Cyprus, Israel and California. It is extracted by cold expression of fresh lemon peel (a distilled oil is also available, but it has an inferior aroma). The expressed oil is pale yellow with a fresh, sharp scent. Its odour effect is uplifting and cooling.

Aromatherapy Uses
Skin care (oily skin), acne, boils, chilblains, cellulite, arthritis, high blood pressure, poor circulation, rheumatic and arthritic aches and pains, sore throat, bronchitis, cararrh, colds and flu, nevous tension and mild depression.

Blending Guide
Top note; moderately high odour intensity.
It blends well with most other oils, including other citrus essences, Roman chamomile, coriander and other spices, cypress, frankincense, juniper, lavender, myrrh, neroli, petitgrain, pine, rose, rosemary, sandalwood, tea tree, ylang-ylang.

CAUTION
Like other citrus oils, expressed lemon oil (but not the steam-distilled version) is phototoxic. Do not apply to skin before exposure to sunlight (or a sunbed). Lemon oil should be used within six to nine months of opening the bottle. The oil may irritate sensitive skin; always use in the lowest recommended concentrations.

Citrus reticulata

Mandarin

Family: *Rutaceae*

A small evergreen tree with glossy leaves produces fragrant white flowers, followed by the fleshy fruit. Native to China, today it is cultivated mainly in the Mediterranean. The oil is extracted by cold expression of the rind of the fruit. It is yellowy-orange with a gentle, sweet citrus scent. Its odour effect is soothing and uplifting.

Aromatherapy Uses
Oily skin conditions, prevention of stretch marks during pregnancy, indigestion, insomnia, nervous tension.

Blending Guide
Top note; very low odour intensity.
Mandarin blends well with other citrus oils, also lavender, petitgrain, neroli, cedarwood, black pepper, coriander, frankincense, rose otto, rose absolute, rosemary, sandalwood, lemongrass, palmarosa, ylang-ylang.

CAUTION
The oil is slightly phototoxic and may cause unsightly pigmentation if applied to skin shortly before exposure to sunlight (or a sunbed). Like most other citrus essences, it has a relatively short shelf-life. Use within six to nine months of opening.

Citrus sinensis

Orange, sweet

Family: *Rutaceae*

This evergreen green tree with glossy leaves produces fragrant white flowers, followed by the fruits. Most of the oil is produced in France, Italy, Israel, Cyprus and the USA, and is extracted by cold expression of the rind of the fruit. An inferior grade essential oil is distilled from the fruit pulp, a by-product of orange juice manufacture. The preferred expressed oil is yellowy-orange with a sweet and refreshing aroma. Its odour effect is cooling, uplifting and cheering.

Aromatherapy Uses
Palpitations, bronchitis, colds and flu, indigestion, mild depression, nervous tension and other stress-related states.

Blending Guide
Top note; medium odour intensity.
Blends well with other citrus essences, clary sage, coriander, ginger, frankincense, geranium, lavender, myrrh, neroli, patchouli, rosemary, spikenard.

CAUTION
Some reports suggest that both the expressed and distilled oils are phototoxic; other studies indicate otherwise. Certainly the oil extracted from the rind of the bitter orange (*C. aurantium* var. *amara*) is much more likely to provoke photosensitivity. Nevertheless, avoid skin applications of sweet orange oil before exposure to sunlight (or a sunbed). Use the oil in the lowest recommended concentrations. Orange oil deteriorates very quickly; use it within six months.

Citrus x paradisi

Grapefruit

Family: *Rutaceae*

A cultivated citrus tree with glossy leaves, fragrant white flowers and large yellow fruits. Most of the oil is produced in California, and is extracted by cold expression of the fresh peel of the fruit. (A lower grade oil can be obtained by steam distillation of the peel and fruit pulp, but this is not recommended for aromatherapy.) The expressed oil is pale or greenish-yellow with a sweet, citrus fragrance. Its odour effect is uplifting and refreshing.

Aromatherapy Uses

Oily skin conditions, colds and flu, mild depression, nervous exhaustion. Reputedly helpful for cellulite, though needs to be used in combination with a good massage.

Blending Guide

Top note; medium odour intensity.
Blends well with other citrus essences, cardamom, coriander, cypress, juniper, lavender, neroli, petitgrain, pine, geranium, rosemary, tea tree.

CAUTION

The expressed oil (but not the steam-distilled whole fruit oil) is slightly phototoxic and must not be applied to skin shortly before exposure to sunlight (or a sunbed) as it may promote unsightly pigmentation. Grapefruit oil, like other citrus essences, has a relatively short shelf-life and must be used within six to nine months of opening.

Commiphora myrrha

Myrrh

Family: *Burseraceae*

The oil is extracted by steam distillation of myrrh 'tears' – little pieces of solidified oleo gum resin – which exude from natural fissures in the bark of this small tree or shrub. The myrrh plant is native to the Middle East, North Africa and Northern India. The oil is a pale amber, slightly viscous substance with a warm, balsamic, 'medicinal' aroma. Its odour effect is head-clearing and warming.

Aromatherapy Uses

Athlete's foot, arthritic pain, chapped and cracked skin, ringworm, wounds, bronchitis, catarrh, coughs, gingivitis, mouth ulcers, sore throat, laryngitis, indigestion, delayed periods outside pregnancy, thrush, colds and flu.

Blending Guide

Base note; very high odour intensity.
Used sparingly, it blends well with citrus oils, cypress, frankincense, juniper berry, lavender, orange, palmarosa, pine, geranium, patchouli, peppermint, ginger, coriander, lemongrass, sandalwood.

CAUTION

It is essential that you purchase the essential oil of myrrh, not myrrh resinoid. The latter is a sticky substance, solidifying with age, captured by means of volatile solvents. Myrrh is also tentatively regarded as an emmenagogue (a substance capable of promoting menstruation), so avoid skin applications during pregnancy.

Coriandrum sativum

Coriander

Family: *Apiaceae (Umbelliferae)*

A strongly aromatic herb with bright green delicate leaves and umbels of lace-like white flowers, followed by a mass of green (turning brown) seeds. Native to Europe and western Asia, although cultivated world-wide. Most of the oil is produced in Eastern Europe. It is extracted by steam distillation of the crushed, ripe seeds. The oil is colourless to pale yellow with a pungent, sweet-spicy, faintly musky aroma. Its odour effect is warming, uplifting and stimulating; a reputed aphrodisiac.

● Aromatherapy Uses

Arthritic and rheumatic pain, muscular aches and pains, facial neuralgia, poor circulation, digestive problems, colds and flu, mental fatigue, nervous exhaustion.

● Blending Guide

Middle note; fairly high odour intensity.
Blends well with other spices, cistus, citrus oils, geranium, rose, cypress, juniper, petitgrain, neroli, pine, frankincense, sandalwood.

Cupressus sempervirens

Cypress

Family: *Cupressaceae*

A tall evergreen tree with slender branches and conical shape. Cypress is native to the Mediterranean. Most of the oil is produced in France, Spain and Morocco. The oil is extracted by steam distillation of the needles, twigs and cones. It is pale greenish-yellow with a fresh, woody balsamic aroma. Although the aroma is also somewhat medicinal, it is often described as pleasantly cooling and calming.

● Aromatherapy Uses

Skin care (oily skin), acne, poor circulation, excessive perspiration, gum disorders, wounds, bronchitis, spasmodic coughs, rheumatism, excessive menstruation, menopausal distress, nervous tension and other stress-related states.

● Blending Guide

Middle to base note; fairly high odour intensity. Blends well with bergamot and other citrus oils, Canadian balsam, clary sage, frankincense, petitgrain, pine, juniper berry, lavender, sweet marjoram, sandalwood.

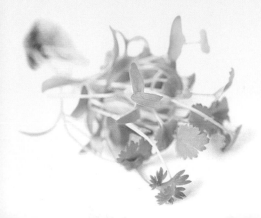

Cymbopogon citratus

Lemongrass, West Indian

Family: *Poaceae (Gramineae)*

Other species: The essence is also extracted from
C. flexuosus, East Indian lemongrass

A fast-growing aromatic grass native to tropical Asia,
although cultivated in other areas. Most of the oil,
whether 'West Indian' or 'East Indian' is produced
in Guatemala and India. It is extracted by steam
distillation of the fresh and partially dried grass, finely
chopped. It is yellow or light amber, with sweet, lemony
top notes and a grassy undertone. Its odour effect is
uplifting and refreshing. Some people find the aroma
quite relaxing, others regard it as a 'wake up' oil.

Aromatherapy Uses
Oily skin conditions, athlete's foot, as an insect
repellent, scabies, muscular aches and pains, poor
circulation, insufficient milk in breastfeeding
mothers, indigestion, fevers, as a fumigant when
infectious illness is around, headaches, nervous
exhaustion and other stress-related states.

Blending Guide
Top to middle note; very high odour intensity. It
blends well with mandarin and other citrus essences,
cardamom, chamomile (Roman and German),
coriander, eucalyptus, geranium, ginger, lavender,
myrrh, palmarosa, patchouli, petitgrain, rosemary.

CAUTION
Lemongrass may irritate sensitive skin. Use in the
lowest recommended concentration of 0.5–1 per
cent. The potential irritant effect is lessened if
blended with an equal quantity of mandarin oil.

Cymbopogon martinii

Palmarosa

Family: *Gramineae*

Native to India, palmarosa is an aromatic grass. It
is closely related to other aromatic grasses such
as lemongrass, citronella and vetiver. Palmarosa is
cultivated in Africa, Indonesia, Madagascar and the
nearby Comoros Islands, where most of the oil is
produced. Captured by steam distillation of the fresh
or dried grass, it is yellowish-green with a strong,
sweet, geranium-like aroma and earthy undertone.
The odour effect is uplifting and energizing.

Aromatherapy Uses
Skin care (especially oily skin), acne, boils,
wounds, loss of appetite, digestive upsets, feverish
conditions, nervous exhaustion and other
stress-related states.

Blending Guide
Middle to base note; high odour intensity.
Palmarosa blends well with cedarwood, citrus
essences, Roman chamomile, clary sage, coriander
and other spice oils, neroli, coriander, geranium,
lavender, lemongrass, patchouli, petitgrain,
sandalwood, vetiver.

Daucus carota

Carrot Seed

Family: *Apiaceae (Umbelliferae)*

A tall evergreeen tree with bluish-green, sword-shaped leaves and creamy-white flowers. The tree is native to Australia and Tasmania and is also cultivated in Spain, Portugal, Brazil, California and China, from where much of the world's supply of eucalyptus oil is produced. The oil is extracted by steam distillation of the leaves and young twigs. It is virtually colourless with a piercing, camphoreous aroma. Its odour effect is head-clearing, mentally stimulating and cooling.

◆ Aromatherapy Uses

General skin care (for revitalizing and toning), arthritis, rheumatism, gout, as a supportive remedy for detoxification purposes, as a restorative during convalescence, indigestion, PMS (may help with fluid retention).

◆ Blending Guide

Middle note; quite high odour intensity.
Blends well with bergamot and other citrus oils, coriander and other spices, cedarwood, Roman chamomile, sweet marjoram, geranium, lavender, rose, ylang-ylang.

Elettaria cardamomum

Cardamom

Family: *Zingiberaceae*

Native to tropical Asia, cardomom is a member of the ginger family. It is a reed-like shrub rising from fleshy rhizomes, producing small yellow flowers which are followed by fruits or seed capsules (the familiar cardomom pods). Most of the oil is produced in India, captured by steam distillation of the dried seeds. It is a colourless to pale yellow liquid, with a sweet, spicy balsamic aroma. Its odour effect is warming, head-clearing and enlivening; a reputed aphrodisiac.

◆ Aromatherapy Uses

Indigestion, colic, flatulence, bad breath, mental fatigue, nervous exhaustion.

◆ Blending Guide

Middle note; extremely high odour intensity.
Blends well with coriander, cedarwood, frankincense, ginger, citrus oils, cistus, rose, geranium, lavender, neroli, ylang-ylang.

◆ CAUTION

A powerful oil, so use in low concentrations of 0.5 per cent.

Eucalyptus globulus

Eucalyptus

Family: *Myrtaceae*

A tall evergreen tree with bluish-green, sword-shaped leaves and creamy-white flowers. Native to Australia and Tasmania, it is also cultivated in Spain, Portugal, Brazil, California and China, from where much of the world's supply of eucalyptus oil is produced. The oil is extracted by steam distillation of the leaves and young twigs. It is virtually colourless with a piercing, camphoric aroma. Its odour effect is head-clearing, mentally stimulating and cooling.

◗ Aromatherapy Uses

Burns, blisters, chickenpox, measles, cold sores, cuts, insect bites and stings, insect repellant, headlice, skin infections, wounds, arthritic pain, muscular aches and pains, sprains, poor circulation, cystitis, hayfever, colds and flu, headaches, neur-algia, mental fatigue, as a fumigant when infectious illness is around.

◗ Blending Guide

Top note; high odour intensity.
Blends well with cedarwood, frankincense, lavender, lemon, tea tree, sweet marjoram, myrrh, peppermint, pine, rosemary.

◗ CAUTION

In skin applications, use in low concentration as it may cause irritation. The oil should not be used on young children.

Helichrysum italicum

Helichrysum

Family: *Asteraceae (Compositae)*

A strongly aromatic herb with clusters of small bright yellow flowers. When dried, the flowers keep their shape and colour – hence the plant is commonly known as 'everlasting' or 'immortelle'. The oil is produced mainly in Italy, France and Spain, and is extracted by steam distillation of the fresh flowers. The oil is pale yellow or reddish with a powerful, rich, honey-like aroma. Its odour effect is warming and energizing.

◗ Aromatherapy Uses

Abscesses, acne, boils, bruises, cuts, inflamed skin conditions, healing scar tissue, muscular aches and pains, rheumatism, sprains, bronchitis, coughs, colds and flu, mild depression, nervous exhaustion and other stress-related conditions.

◗ Blending Guide

Middle to base note; high odour intensity.
Used sparingly, it blends well with chamomile (German and Roman), lemon and other citrus oils, cistus, lavender, geranium, clary sage, rose.

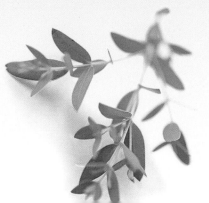

Hypericum perforatum

Hypericum/St John's wort

Family: Hypericaceae

NB: The product described here is not an essential oil, but an infused or macerated oil.

A wild herb native to Europe and North America, with vibrant yellow, star-shaped flowers and narrow leaves dotted with tiny oil glands. Although the plant yields an essential oil, very few distillers are producing it. Aromatherapists usually employ the infused oil, obtained by macerating the crushed flowering tops in vegetable oil (usually sunflower or olive). The resulting oil is ruby-red due to the pigment hypericum.

Aromatherapy Uses
An anti-inflammatory oil for wounds, bruises, muscular aches and pains, rheumatic pain, sciatica.

Blending Guide
Mixed 50:50 with infused calendula oil, its skin-healing properties are enhanced. For aches and pains, its properties can be enhanced with a little rosemary, lavender or sweet marjoram essential oil. The usual ratio is one drop of essential oil per 15–20ml hypericum oil.

CAUTION
Hypericum heightens the skin's sensitivity to sunlight, so do not apply shortly before sunbathing. There is some evidence that St John's wort, when taken internally, may sometimes cause allergic reactions.

Juniperus communis

Juniper Berry

Family: Cupressaceae

A small, evergreen conifer tree, with bluish-green needles and bluish-black berries. The tree is native to North America, Europe, northern Asia and Japan. The highest grade oil is extracted by steam distillation of the fruits rather than from the fermented berries. An oil is also extracted from the needles and wood and labelled 'Juniper Needle'. Aromatherapists favour oil captured from virgin berries. The aroma of the best juniper berry oil is fresh and woody with a hint of pepper. Its odour effect is uplifting, yet warming and calming; a reputed aphrodisiac.

Aromatherapy Uses
Skin and hair care (oily), acne, haemorrhoids, wounds, cellulite, arthritic and rheumatic complaints, muscular aches, delayed or painful menstruation, cystitis, PMS, nervous tension and other stresses.

Blending Guide
Middle note; fairly high odour intensity. Blends well with citrus oils, Canadian balsam, cedarwood, cypress, frankincense, geranium, lavender, neroli, petitgrain, pine, rosemary, sandalwood, tea tree, vetiver.

CAUTION
Avoid skin applications during pregnancy as the oil may stimulate the uterus. This method is also best avoided by people with kidney disease. Do not use on young children. Only buy from a reputable supplier, for although it can be a skin irritant, this may be because it is often adulterated with turpentine.

Juniperus virginiana

Cedarwood, Virginian

Family: *Cupressaceae*

An evergreen conifer tree native to eastern and central North America, its oil is extracted by steam distillation of the wood, stumps and sawdust. A yellowish amber, viscous liquid with a sweet, woody aroma which improves with age. Its odour effect is head-clearing and calming; a reputed aphrodisiac.

Aromatherapy Uses
Acne, oily skin, dandruff, fungal infections, arthritis, rheumatism, bronchitis, coughs, sinusitis, emotional symptoms of PMS, delayed menstruation outside pregnancy, nervous tension and other stress-related disorders. .

Blending Guide
Middle to base note; low odour intensity.
Blends well with bergamot, Canadian balsam, clary sage, cypress, frankincense, geranium, juniper berry, lemon, neroli, palmarosa, petitgrain, pine, rose, rosemary, sandalwood, vetiver, ylang-ylang.

CAUTION
Avoid during pregnancy. May irritate sensitive skin, so use in the lowest recommended concentrations.

Lavandula angustifolia

Lavender

Family: *Lamiaceae (Labiatae)*

An evergreen, woody shrub producing abundant spikes of bluish-mauve flowers, native to the Medi-terranean. Extracted by steam distillation of the flowering tops, this pale-yellow oil has a sweet floral-herbaceous fragrance. Its odour effect is uplifting, calming and refreshing.

Aromatherapy Uses
Skin care (most skin types), acne, athlete's foot, boils, bruises, inflamed skin, dandruff, burns, chilblains, ringworm, scabies, insect bites, insect repellent, earache, coughs, colds and flu, catarrh, laryngitis, muscular aches, rheumatic pain, nausea, colic, cystitis, painful menstruation, mild depression, headache, insomnia, migraine, PMS, nervous tension and other stress-related states.

Blending Guide
Middle note; medium odour intensity.
Blends well with most other essences, especially cedarwood, chamomile (Roman and German), cistus, clary sage, coriander, cypress, frankincense, geranium, juniper berry, neroli, rose, petitgrain, pine, vetiver.

CAUTION
Although regarded as a non-irritant, it is possible to be skin-sensitive to one brand of lavender and not to another, even though both types may be labelled *L. angustifolia*. This may suggest that the oil has been adulterated or has oxidized. Only buy from a reputable supplier and use within one year.

Matricaria recutica

Chamomile, German

Family. *Asteraceae (Compositae)*

A strongly aromatic herb with delicate feathery leaves and simple daisy-like white flowers. The plant is native to Europe and north and west Asia. It is captured by steam distillation of the flower heads. The oil is inky-blue and viscous with a sweetish, warm-herbaceous aroma. Its odour effect is warming and soothing.

◖ Aromatherapy Uses

Skin care (most skin types including sensitive), skin rashes, boils, burns, wounds, chilblains, earache, insect bites and stings, inflammation and swelling (caused by injury), muscular aches, arthritic and rheumatic pain, sprains and strains, neuralgia, teething pain, toothache, indigestion, painful or heavy periods, headache, migraine, insomnia, PMS, nervous tension and other stress-related states.

◖ Blending Guide

Middle note; very high odour intensity.
Blends well with bergamot and other citrus oils, rose, lavender, geranium, neroli, helichrysum, sweet marjoram, clary sage, cistus.

◖ CAUTION

German chamomile has a high concentration of chamazulene, which is responsible for its deep blue colour, and for its excellent anti-inflammatory properties. However, when treating inflamed skin conditions, always use the oil in the lowest recommended concentrations of 0.5–1 per cent, otherwise it may exacerbate the condition.

Melaleuca alternifolia

Tea tree

Family: *Myrtaceae*

This small tree or shrub with needle-like leaves and bottlebrush-like yellow flowers is native to Australia, where the world's supply of tea tree oil is produced. The oil is extracted by steam distillation of the leaves and twigs. It is pale yellow with a strong, spicy-camphoric aroma. The odour effect is energizing and head-clearing.

◖ Aromatherapy Uses

Acne, athlete's foot, abscesses, cold sores, dandruff, rashes, ringworm, burns, wounds, insect bites and stings, colds and flu, catarrh, coughs, verruca, thrush, cystitis, fevers, as a fumigant when infectious illness is around.

◖ Blending Guide

Top note; very high odour intensity.
Used sparingly, it blends well with cypress, clary sage, coriander, eucalyptus, lemon and other citrus oils, lavender, geranium, juniper berry, marjoram, pine, rosemary.

◖ CAUTION

There are many reports of minor skin reactions caused by continuous use of tea tree. Do not use the oil neat or in high concentration for more than six weeks.

Mentha piperita

Peppermint

Family: *Lamiaceae*

A spreading herb with dark green leaves and reddish-violet flowers. Native to the Mediterranean and western Asia, most of the world's supply of peppermint oil is produced in the USA. Captured by steam distillation of the flowering tops, it is pale yellow with a fresh, piercing, minty aroma. Its odour effect is awakening, cooling and head-clearing.

Aromatherapy Uses

Bruises, sprains and strains, swelling, ringworm, scabies, toothache, neuralgia, muscular aches, bronchitis, bad breath, sinusitis, spasmodic cough, colic, indigestion, irritable bowel syndrome (taken internally in the form of peppermint capsules according to the maker's instructions), flatulence, mouth ulcers, nausea, feverish conditions, colds and flu, fainting, headache, mental fatigue, migraine.

Blending Guide

Top note; very high odour intensity.
Used sparingly, it blends well with bergamot, clary sage, eucalyptus, lavender, lemon, sweet marjoram, rosemary, sandalwood.

CAUTION

For skin applications, use in the lowest recommended concentrations of 0.5–1 per cent. It is also advisable to avoid skin applications during pregnancy. Do not use on babies and young children, as it may cause breathing problems due to its high menthol content.

Myrtus communis

Myrtle

Family: *Myrtaceae*

A small tree with small, sharp-pointed leaves and white flowers, followed by small black berries. Native to North Africa, but cultivated extensively in the Mediterranean. The oil varies in its biochemical composition, depending on the country of origin. For therapeutic purposes the best quality is produced in Corsica. Extracted by steam distillation of the leaves and twigs, the Corsican oil has a brilliant green hue, whereas the North African variety generally has a reddish tint. The aroma is fresh and camphoric, similar to eucalyptus but sweeter and less piercing. Its odour effect is head-clearing, uplifting and refreshing.

Aromatherapy Uses

Skin care (oily), acne, bronchitis, catarrh, coughs, colds and flu, as a fumigant when infectious illness is around, and for stress-related states. Much safer than eucalyptus for childrens' respiratory ailments.

Blending Guide

Top to middle note; moderately high odour intensity.
Blends well with bergamot, grapefruit, lemon, clary sage, lemon, lavender, cardamom, ginger, coriander.

Nardostachys jatamansi

Spikenard

Family: *Valerianaceae*

A tender aromatic herb with pungent rhizomes ('roots'). The plant is native to the mountainous regions of northern India, and also China and Japan. However, most of the world's supply of oil is produced in Europe and the USA. It is captured by steam distillation of the imported dried rhizomes. The oil is pale yellow or amber-coloured with a heavy, sweet and woody, spice and musk aroma. Its odour effect is calming, soothing and 'grounding'.

◆ Aromatherapy Uses
Mainly for stress-related conditions, such as nervous indigestion, anxiety and insomnia.

◆ Blending Guide
Base note; extremely high odour intensity.
Used sparingly, it blends well with bergamot and other citrus oils, clary sage, cistus, frankincense, lavender, neroli, patchouli, petitgrain, pine, vetiver, coriander, rose, sandalwood.

Origanum majorana

Marjoram, sweet

Family: *Lamiaceae (Labiatae)*

A tender bushy herb with dark-green oval leaves and small greyish-white flowers produced in clusters or 'knots'. The plant is native to the Mediterranean, but cultivated worldwide. Most of the oil is produced in France, North Africa and Eastern Europe, and extracted by steam distillation of the dried flowering herb. Light amber with a woody, camphoric aroma, its odour effect is warming and calming; a reputed anaphrodisiac, it apparently quells sexual desire.

◆ Aromatherapy Uses
Chilblains, bruises, arthritic and rheumatic pain, muscular aches, sprains and strains, bronchitis, coughs, colic, constipation, flatulence, delayed periods, painful menstruation, PMS, colds and flu, headache, high blood pressure, insomnia, migraine, nervous tension and other stress-related states.

◆ Blending Guide
Middle note; medium odour intensity.
It blends well with bergamot, carrot seed, cedarwood, cypress, chamomile (Roman and German), eucalyptus, juniper berry, lavender, rosemary, tea tree.

◆ CAUTION
Avoid skin applications during pregnancy, as the oil has a reputation for promoting menstruation. Do not confuse sweet marjoram with so-called Spanish marjoram (*Thymus mastichina*) which is actually a species of thyme. Spanish marjoram is not recommended for home use as it is a skin irritant.

Pelargonium graveolens

Geranium

Family: *Geraniaceae*

Other species: There are a number of oil-producing pelargoniums, including *P. odorantissimum*, *P. roseum*, *P. radens*, and various hybrid varieties.

A spreading shrub with pointed leaves, serrated at the edges, and small rose-pink flowers. The plant is native to South Africa. The oil is extracted by steam distillation of the leaves, stalks and flowers. It is olive-green with a piercingly sweet and rosy scent. Bourbon geranium, which has the best aroma, also emits a background nuance of mint. Geranium's odour effect is refreshing and uplifting. Intriguingly, it can be relaxing for some people and enlivening for others.

Aromatherapy Uses
Skin care (most skin types), burns, headlice, ringworm, neuralgia, poor circulation, engorgement of the breasts in breastfeeding mothers, menopausal distress, PMS, nervous tension, mild depression and other stress-related states.

Blending Guide
Middle note; high odour intensity.
Blends well with many other oils, especially coriander, Roman chamomile, citrus essences, neroli, patchouli, petitgrain, rosemary, sandalwood, vetiver, ylang-ylang.

CAUTION
A highly odoriferous oil, so use in the lowest recommended concentrations.

Pinus sylvestris

Pine, Scots

Family: *Pinaceae*

A tall evergreen conifer tree native to northern Europe. The oil is captured by steam distillation of the pine needles. An inferior grade oil is extracted from the cones, twigs and wood chippings, but this is not recommended for aromatherapy. The best quality oil is colourless to pale yellow. It has a strong, dry, turpentine-like aroma. Its odour effect is refreshing, cooling and restorative.

Aromatherapy Uses
Cuts and abrasions, wounds, headlice, scabies, excessive perspiration, arthritic and rheumatic pain, gout, muscular aches and pains, poor circulation, bronchitis, catarrh, colds and flu, coughs, sinusitis, sore throat, cystitis, neuralgia, nervous exhaustion and other stress-related states.

Blending Guide
Top to middle note; high odour intensity.
Blends well with bergamot and other citrus oils, Canadian balsam, cedarwood, cypress, eucalyptus, frankincense, juniper, lavender, rosemary, tea tree, eucalyptus, spikenard, sweet marjoram.

CAUTION
Pine oil must be used within one year of opening, An aged or oxidized oil may cause skin irritation. Always use the lowest recommended concentration. Direct skin applications are not advisable for children or for anyone else with sensitive skin.

Piper nigrum

Black Pepper

Family: *Piperaceae*

Black pepper is a large twining plant or vine, native to India, but now extensively cultivated in Malaysia, China and Madagasgar. The oil is extracted by steam distillation of the dried fruits (peppercorns). It is a pale greenish-yellow with a hot, spicy, piquant aroma. Its odour effect is stimulating and warming; a reputed aphrodisiac.

Aromatherapy Uses
Poor circulation, poor muscle tone, muscular aches and pains, rheumatic pain, sprains, loss of appetite after illness, nausea, colds and flu, lethargy, mental fatigue.

Blending Guide
Middle to base note; high odour intensity. Blends well with other spices, citrus essences, frankincense, lavender, geranium, rose, ylang-ylang, rosemary, sandalwood.

CAUTION
An irritant when used in concentration. For skin applications, use in the lowest recommended concentrations of one per cent or less. Applications of the oil are best avoided during the first trimester of pregnancy.

Pogostemon cablin

Patchouli

Family: *Lamiaceae (Labiatae)*

A herbaceous plant with soft, 'furry' leaves and white flowers tinged with purple. Patchouli is native to Malaysia, but cultivated in India, China and South America. The oil is extracted by steam distillation of the dried fermented leaves. It is a dark-amber viscous liquid with an extremely tenacious, earthy-musky aroma, which becomes sweeter as the harsh top notes begin to wane. Unlike most other essential oils, the scent of patchouli improves with age. Its odour effect is warming and restorative; a reputed aphrodisiac.

Aromatherapy Uses
Skin and hair care (especially oily skin and scalp conditions), abscesses, acne, athlete's foot, bed sores, cracked and sore skin, dandruff, as an insect repellent, wounds, mild depression, nervous exhaustion and other stress-related states.

Blending Guide
Base note; extremely high odour intensity. Used sparingly, it blends well with bergamot and other citrus essences, cedarwood, clary sage, lavender, myrrh, geranium, palmarosa, petitgrain, rose, spikenard, neroli, sandalwood, vetiver.

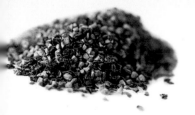

Rosa damascena

Rose otto

Family: *Rosaceae*

NB: A solvent-extracted rose absolute (a reddish-orange liquid) is also widely available, but the distilled rose otto is preferable for therapeutic use.

A small, prickly shrub with pink, intensely fragrant blooms. The oil is captured by steam distillation of the fresh petals. Rosewater (or hydrolat or hydrosol) is produced as a by-product. The essential oil is virtually colourless and becomes semi-solid at cool temperatures. The aroma is rich, sweet and mellow with a hint of spice and vanilla. The odour effect is warming, soothing and heady; a reputed aphrodisiac.

◖ Aromatherapy Uses
Skin care (especially mature), conjunctivitis (rosewater only), thread veins, inflamed skin, palpitations, hay fever, poor circulation, coughs, cold sores, irregular or heavy periods, PMS, mild depression, insomnia, headaches and nervous tension. Rosewater is used mainly as a gentle skin toner.

◖ Blending Guide
Middle note; high odour intensity.
Rose otto blends well with most other essences, especially neroli, Roman chamomile, lavender, bergamot and other citrus oils, coriander and other spice oils, geranium, helichrysum, bergamot, clary sage, sandalwood, spikenard, patchouli.

◖ CAUTION
On skin, use in low concentration as it may cause irritation. Do not use on young children.

Rosmarinus officinalis

Rosemary

Family: *Lamiaceae (Labiatae)*

A shrubby evergreen bush with silvery-green needle-shaped leaves and pale blue flowers. Native to the Mediterranean, though now cultivated worldwide. Most of the oil is produced in France, Spain and Tunisia. It is extracted by steam distillation of the flowering tops. Inferior oils are distilled from the whole plant. The best oil is pale yellow with a woody-balsamic, camphoric aroma. Lower quality oils are more highly camphoric (like eucalyptus), and somewhat harsh. The odour effect is head-clearing, warming and restorative.

◖ Aromatherapy Uses
Skin and hair care (oily), dandruff, to promote growth of healthy hair, headlice, as an insect repellent, scabies, colds and flu, bronchitis, coughs, muscular aches and pains, arthritic and rheumatic pain, poor circulation, painful menstruation, headaches, mental fatigue, neuralgia, depression, nervous exhaustion and other stress-related states.

◖ Blending Guide
Top to middle note; moderately high odour intensity. Blends well with cedarwood, coriander and other spice oils, citrus essences, frankincense, geranium, lemongrass, lavender, peppermint, petitgrain, pine.

◖ CAUTION
Avoid skin applications during pregnancy. There is a remote chance that the oil may trigger an epileptic seizure in those predisposed to the condition.

Salvia sclarea

Clary sage

Family: *Lamiaceae (Labiatae)*

A shrubby, highly aromatic herb with spikes of white, violet or pink flowers. Clary sage is native to the Mediterranean, but cultivated worldwide. Most of the oil is produced in France and Morocco. It is extracted by steam distillation of the flowering tops and leaves. It is colourless to pale yellow, with a sweetly herbaceous, slightly floral scent. Its odour effect is uplifting and relaxing; a reputed aphrodisiac.

◗ Aromatherapy Uses

High blood pressure, muscular aches, throat infections, coughs, migraine, labour pain and to facilitate birth, irregular menstruation, PMS, menopausal distress, mild depression and nervous tension.

◗ Blending Guide

Top to middle note; fairly high odour intensity.
Clary sage blends well with most oils, especially bergamot, cedarwood, juniper berry, lavender, neroli, petitgrain, pine, frankincense, vetiver.

◗ CAUTION

Avoid skin applications during pregnancy (except during labour). Although the oil may cause excessive drowsiness when used immediately before or after drinking alcohol, clary may not be especially potent in this respect. Any form of relaxing massage will intensify the effects of alcohol.

Santalum album

Sandalwood

Family: *Santalaceae*

This semi-parasitic tree grows on the roots of neighbouring trees during the first seven years of its life and is native to tropical Asia. Today, most of the oil is produced in Indonesia. It is captured by steam distillation of the roots and heartwood of the tree. Sandalwood oil is pale yellow and viscous, with a soft, sweet-woody, balsamic aroma of excellent tenacity. Its odour effect is usually perceived as soothing and deeply relaxing; reputedly aphrodisiac.

◗ Aromatherapy Uses

Skin care (acne, dry, oily), bronchitis, catarrh, coughs, laryngitis, sore throat, diarrhoea, nausea, cystitis, mild depression, insomnia, nervous tension and other stress-related states.

◗ Blending Guide

Base note; low odour intensity.
Blends well with many other oils, especially rose, ylang-ylang, lavender, coriander and other spices, bergamot, clary sage, geranium, cistus, vetiver, patchouli, frankincense, spikenard, pine, myrrh.

◗ CAUTION

Due to its high price and scarcity, sandalwood oil is especially vulnerable to adulteration. It is also one of the easiest aromatics to replicate in the laboratory Occasionally, the oil known as West Indian sandalwood (*Amyris balsamifera*) is sold as an inexpensive alternative to genuine sandalwood. West Indian sandalwood oil (also commonly known as Amyris) bears no relation to true sandalwood oil.

Vetiveria zizanioides

Vetiver

Family: *Poaceae (Gramineae)*

A tall grass with unscented leaves, but highly aromatic roots. The plant is a close relative of other aromatic grasses such as lemongrass and palmarosa. Native to southern India, Indonesia and Sri Lanka, but also cultivated in other regions. The highest quality oil is obtained from Réunion and the Comoros Islands. It is extracted by steam distillation of the dried and chopped roots. The oil is dark brown and viscous with a highly tenacious, earthy, molasses-like aroma. The fragrance improves as the oil ages. Its odour effect is calming and warming; a reputed aphrodisiac.

◢ Aromatherapy Uses

Skin care (oily), acne, arthritic and rheumatic pain, muscular aches and pains, poor circulation, insomnia, stress-related light-headedness (a good 'grounding' essence), PMS, mild depression, nervous exhaustion and other stress-related states.

◢ Blending Guide

Base note; very high odour intensity. Used sparingly, vetiver blends well with clary sage, cedarwood, citrus oils, lavender, patchouli, petitgrain, neroli, rose, sandalwood, ylang-ylang.

Zingiber officinalis

Ginger

Family: *Zingiber officinale*

This tall reed-like plant stems from tuberous rhizomes. Ginger is native to southern Asia and is cultivated commercially in the West Indies and Africa. Most of the oil is distilled in China and India by steam distillation of the dried, ground rhizomes or 'roots'. It is pale amber with a pungent, warm and spicy aroma. However, it lacks the fruity top note found in the raw plant material because the process of distillation alters its original chemical structure. The odour effect is warming and stimulating; a reputed aphrodisiac.

◢ Aromatherapy Uses

Arthritic and rheumatic pain, muscular aches and pains, poor circulation, catarrh, coughs, sore throat, diarrhoea, colic, indigestion, loss of appetite after illness, nausea, travel sickness, colds and flu, mental fatigue, nervous exhaustion and as a fumigant when infectious illness is around.

◢ Blending Guide

Middle to base note; extremely high odour intensity. Used sparingly, ginger blends well with cedarwood, coriander and other spices, citrus essences, frankincense, neroli, patchouli, petitgrain, rose, sandalwood, vetiver, ylang-ylang.

◢ CAUTION

The oil may irritate sensitive skin. Use in the lowest recommended concentrations of 0.5–1 per cent.

A Quick Guide to Essential Oils for Specific Ailments

Treatment strategies for many of the ailments can be found from pages 30–92. For general advice on preparing essential oils for various applications, see Aromatherapy Foundations, page 14.

◗ Abscess
Chamomile (Roman or German), eucalyptus, helichrysum, lavender, lemon, tea tree.

◗ Acne
Cedarwood (Virginian or Atlas), chamomile (German or Roman), frankincense, geranium, helichrysum, juniper berry, lavender, lemongrass, myrtle, palmarosa, patchouli, rosemary, sandalwood, tea tree, vetiver. Also, calendula tincture diluted 1:6 in water.

◗ Anxiety
Bergamot, frankincense, juniper berry, lavender, neroli, petitgrain, spikenard, ylang-ylang.

◗ Arthritis and Rheumatism
Black pepper, carrot seed, cedarwood (Virginian or Atlas), chamomile (German or Roman), coriander, cypress, eucalyptus, frankincense, ginger, helichrysum, juniper berry, lavender, lemon, sweet marjoram, myrrh, Scots pine, rosemary, vetiver.

◗ Athlete's Foot
Cedarwood (Virginian or Atlas), eucalyptus, lavender, lemon, lemongrass, myrrh, patchouli, tea tree. Also, calendula oil or tincture. Tincture is best diluted 1:3 in water.

◗ Boils
Chamomile (German or Roman), eucalyptus, helichrysum, lavender, lemon, tea tree. Also, calendula tincture diltued 1:4 in water.

◗ Bronchitis
Canadian balsam, cedarwood (Virginian or Atlas), cistus, cypress, eucalyptus, frankincense, helichrysum, lavender, lemon, myrrh, myrtle, orange, peppermint, rosemary, sandalwood, Scots pine, sweet marjoram, tea tree.

◗ Bruises
Geranium, sweet marjoram, lavender.

◗ Burns and Scalds (including sunburn)
Canadian balsam, chamomile (German or Roman), eucalyptus, geranium, helichrysum, lavender, tea tree. Also, hypericum and calendula tincture (mixed 50:50) diluted 1:6 in water.

◗ Catarrh
Black pepper, Canadian balsam, cedarwood (Virginian and Atlas), eucalyptus, frankincense, ginger, peppermint, myrrh, myrtle, sandalwood, Scots pine, tea tree.

◗ Cellulite
Cypress, geranium, grapefruit, juniper berry, lemon, rosemary.

◗ Chapped and Cracked Skin
German chamomile, myrrh, patchouli, sandalwood. Also, macerated calendula oil.

Chilblains

Back pepper, chamomile (German or Roman), lemon, sweet marjoram.

Circulation, Sluggish

Black pepper, coriander, cypress, eucalyptus, geranium, ginger, lemon, lemongrass, neroli, rose otto, rosemary, Scots pine.

Colds and Flu

Bergamot, cistus, coriander, eucalyptus, frankincense, ginger, grapefruit, helichrysum, juniper berry, lavender, lemon, lime, myrtle, orange, peppermint, rosemary, Scots pine, sweet marjoram, tea tree.

Cold Sores

Eucalyptus, tea tree. Also, calendula and St John's wort/hypericum tincture blended 50:50, diluted 1:3 in water.

Coughs

Black pepper, Canadian balsam, cedarwood (Atlas), cistus, clary sage, cypress, eucalyptus, frankincense, ginger, helichrysum, peppermint, myrrh, myrtle, rose otto, rosemary, sandalwood, sweet marjoram, tea tree.

Cuts, Grazes and Wounds

Canadian balsam, chamomile (German and Roman), cypress, eucalyptus, frankincense, lemon, geranium, lavender. Also, calendula and St John's wort/hypericum tincture (blended 50:50) diluted 1:6 in water.

Dandruff

Cedarwood (Virginian or Atlas), eucalyptus, lavender, patchouli, rosemary, tea tree.

Depression (including post-natal)

Bergamot (and other citrus oils), Canadian balsam, clary sage, frankincense, geranium, helichrysum, lavender, neroli, rosemary, rose otto, sandalwood, vetiver.

Eczema

Home treatment with essential oils is not recommended for this condition (reasons are given on page 51). Itching and inflammation may be eased with calendula tincture incorporated into a cream base at a ratio of 10ml tincture to 30ml base. Alternatively apply calendula tincture diluted 1:8 with water.

Fatigue and Nervous Exhaustion

Bergamot (and other citrus oils), coriander, geranium, ginger, juniper berry, peppermint, lavender, palmarosa, peppermint, rose otto, rosemary, Scots pine, sweet marjoram.

Gum Infections
(including gingivitis)

Bergamot, clary sage, cypress, lemon, myrrh. Also, calendula tincture diluted 1:6 with water and used as a mouthwash.

Haemorrhoids/Piles

Cypress, frankincense, geranium, juniper berry, myrrh, myrtle. Also, distilled witch-hazel applied directly.

Hayfever

Chamomile (German), eucalyptus, lavender, peppermint, rose otto, Scots pine.

Headache

Chamomile (German and Roman), clary sage, eucalyptus, lavender, lemongrass, peppermint, rose otto, rosemary, sweet marjoram.

Headlice

Eucalyptus, geranium, lavender, rosemary.

Indigestion, Flatulence and Heartburn

Black pepper (specifically heartburn), cardamom (including heartburn), carrot seed, chamomile (German or Roman), clary sage, coriander, ginger, lavender, lemongrass, neroli, peppermint, petitgrain, spikenard (nervous indigestion), sweet marjoram.

Insect Bites and Stings

Cedarwood (Virginian), chamomile (German or Roman), eucalyptus, lavender, tea tree. Also, calendula tincture diluted 1:3 with water.

Insect Repellent

Bergamot, cedarwood (Virginian), cypress, eucalyptus, geranium, lavender, lemongrass, patchouli, rosemary.

Insomnia

Chamomile (German and Roman), clary sage, lavender, mandarin, neroli, petitgrain, rose otto, sandalwood, spikenard, sweet marjoram, vetiver.

Irritable Bowel Syndrome

Peppermint (taken by mouth in the form of peppermint oil capsules). See also Anxiety, Stress.

Laryngitis/hoarseness

Clary sage, lemon, eucalyptus, frankincense, lavender, myrrh, sandalwood.

Menopausal Problems

Hot flushes and night sweats: Clary sage, cypress. See also Menstrual Problems, Anxiety, Depression, Stress.

Menstrual Problems

AMENORRHOEA/LOSS OF MENSTRUATION: Carrot seed, clary sage, juniper berry, myrrh, rose otto, sweet marjoram. DYSMENORRHOEA/PAINFUL MENSTRUATION: Carrot seed, chamomile (German or Roman), clary sage, cypress, frankincense, juniper berry, lavender, rose otto, rosemary, sweet marjoram.
MENORRHAGIA/EXCESSIVE MENSTRUATION: Chamomile (German and Roman), cypress, frankincense, rose otto.

Mental Fatigue

Cardamom, coriander, eucalyptus, geranium, lavender, lemon, lime, lemongrass, myrtle, peppermint, Scots pine, rosemary.

Migraine

Chamomile (German or Roman), clary sage, coriander, lavender, peppermint, spikenard, sweet marjoram.

Mouth Ulcers

German chamomile, myrrh, peppermint, tea tree. Also, calendula tincture diluted 1:6 with water and used as a mouthwash.

Muscular Aches and Pains

Black pepper, chamomile, clary sage, coriander, eucalyptus, frankincense, ginger, helichrysum, lavender, lemongrass, sweet marjoram, peppermint, Scots pine, rosemary, vetiver.

Nausea and Vomiting

Black pepper, cardamom, chamomile (German or Roman), coriander, ginger, lavender, peppermint, rose otto, sandalwood.

Palpitations

Lavender, neroli, orange, petitgrain, rose otto, ylang-ylang.

Pre-Menstrual Syndrome (PMS)

EMOTIONAL UPS AND DOWNS: Bergamot, Roman chamomile, clary sage, frankincense, geranium, lavender neroli, rose otto, ylang-ylang (see also Anxiety, Depression, Stress).

FLUID RETENTION: Carrot seed, cypress, geranuim, grapefruit, lavender, juniper berry, rosemary.

Rashes (including nappy rash)

Chamomile (German). Also, calendula and St John's wort/hypericum (macerated oil or tincture) mixed 50:50. Tincture is best incorporated into a cream or ointment base at a ratio of 10ml tincture to 30g base.

Ringworm

Geranium, lavender, myrrh, peppermint, tea tree. Also, calendula tincture incorporated into a cream or ointment base at a ratio of 10ml tincture to 20g base.

Seasonal Affective Disorder (SAD)

See Depression.

Sinusitis

Cistus, eucalyptus, ginger, peppermint, Scots pine, tea tree.

Skin Care, General

COMBINATION SKIN (dry and oily patches): Lavender, frankincense. Also, calendula tincture with a cream or lotion base at a ratio of 10ml tincture to 40g base.

DRY SKIN: Chamomile (German and Roman), lavender, sandalwood and macerated calendula oil.

Sensitive skin: Calendula (macerated oil or tincture). Tincture to be incorporated into cream or ointment base at a ratio of 5ml tincture to 25g base.

OILY SKIN: Carrot seed, cypress, geranium, juniper berry, lemon, lemongrass, myrtle, palmarosa, patchouli, rose otto, rosemary, sandalwood, tea tree, vetiver. Also, calendula tincture incorporated into a lotion base at a ratio of 10ml tincture to 40g base.

Sore, Cracked Nipples

Chamomile (German). Also, calendula and St John's wort/hypericum (macerated oil or tincture) mixed 50:50. Tincture to be incorporated in a cream or ointment base at a ratio of 10ml tincture to 30g base.

Sore Throat

Bergamot, Canadian balsam, clary sage, eucalyptus, geranium, ginger, lavender, myrrh, myrtle, sandalwood, Scots pine, tea tree.

Spots

Lavender, tea tree. Also, calendula tincture diluted 1:3 with water.

Sprains and Strains

Black pepper, chamomile (German and Roman), eucalyptus, ginger, helichrysum, lavender, rosemary, Scots pine, sweet marjoram, vetiver.

Stress

Canadian balsam, bergamot (and other citrus oils), cedarwood (Virginian or Atlas), chamomile (German or Roman), clary sage, cypress, frankincense, geranium, helichrysum, juniper berry, lavender, lemongrass, neroli, palmarosa, patchouli, petitgrain, rose otto, rosemary, sandalwood, Scots pine, spikenard, sweet marjoram, vetiver, ylang-ylang.

Stretch Marks (preventative treatment)

Frankincense, lavender, mandarin, neroli, palmarosa, patchouli, sandalwood, spikenard. Also, calendula (macerated oil or tincture). Tincture should be incorporated into a cream or ointment base at a ratio of 10ml tincture to 40g base.

Varicose Veins

Cypress, frankincense, geranium, juniper berry, myrrh, myrtle. Also, distilled witch-hazel applied directly.

Useful Addresses

UK

For lists of accredited suppliers of essential oils:

The Essential Oil Trade Association
61 Clinton Lane
Kenilworth
Warwickshire
CV8 1AS
Tel: 01926 512001
Fax: 01676 540777
www.eota.org

For lists of accredited aromatherapists and training courses:

International Federation of Aromatherapists
182 Chiswick High Road
London
W4 1PP
Tel: 020 8742 2605
Fax: 020 8742 2606
www.int-fed-aromatherapy.co.uk

For a mail order catalogue of guaranteed certified organic essential oils (this French company supplies the UK and other parts of Europe):

Florial France
42 Chemin des Aubepines,
06130 Grasse
France
Tel: 33 493 778819
Fax: 33 493 778878
Email: info@florial.com

USA

For lists of accredited aromatherapists, training schools and essential oil suppliers:

National Association for Holistic Aromatherapy
Suite 206, 2000 Second Avenue
Seattle
WA 98121
Tel: 206 256 0741
Fax: 206 770 5915
Email: info@naha.org
www.naha.org

AUSTRALIA

For lists of accredited aromatherapists and training courses:

International Federation of Aromatherapists
P.O. Box 305
Doncaster
Victoria 3108
Tel: 411 256049

For essential oils:

Pure Scents
P.O. Box 490
Boronia
Victoria 3155
Tel: 1800 880869
Fax: 1800 880168
Email: info@purescents.com.au
www.purescents.com.au

Suggested Reading

NUTRITION

Edgson, V. and Marber, I., *The Food Doctor – Healing Foods for Mind and Body*, (Collins and Brown, 1999)

HERBAL MEDICINE, FLOWER ESSENCES AND AROMATHERAPY

Wildwood, C., *The Encyclopedia of Healing Plants*, (Piatkus, 1999)

MEDITATION AND STRESS SURVIVAL TECHNIQUES

Wildwood, C., *Natural Healing – Practical Ways to Find Wellbeing and Inspiration*, (Piatkus, 2000)

ESSENTIAL OILS

Lawless, J., *Encyclopedia of Essential Oils*, (Element Books, 1992)

AROMATHERAPY AND MASSAGE

Wildwood, C., *Encyclopedia of Aromatherapy*, (Bloomsbury, 1996 – published in the USA by Healing Arts Press)

Index

Acknowledgements

Thanks to Clare Currie and Emma Baxter for their valuable editorial advice and for soothing the waters when the going got rough! To Claire Graham for designing the book so beautifully and also to Sian Irvine for taking the photographs that appear throughout the book.